YOGA
FOR
CHILDREN

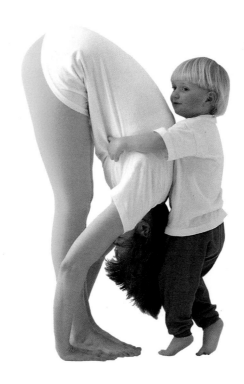

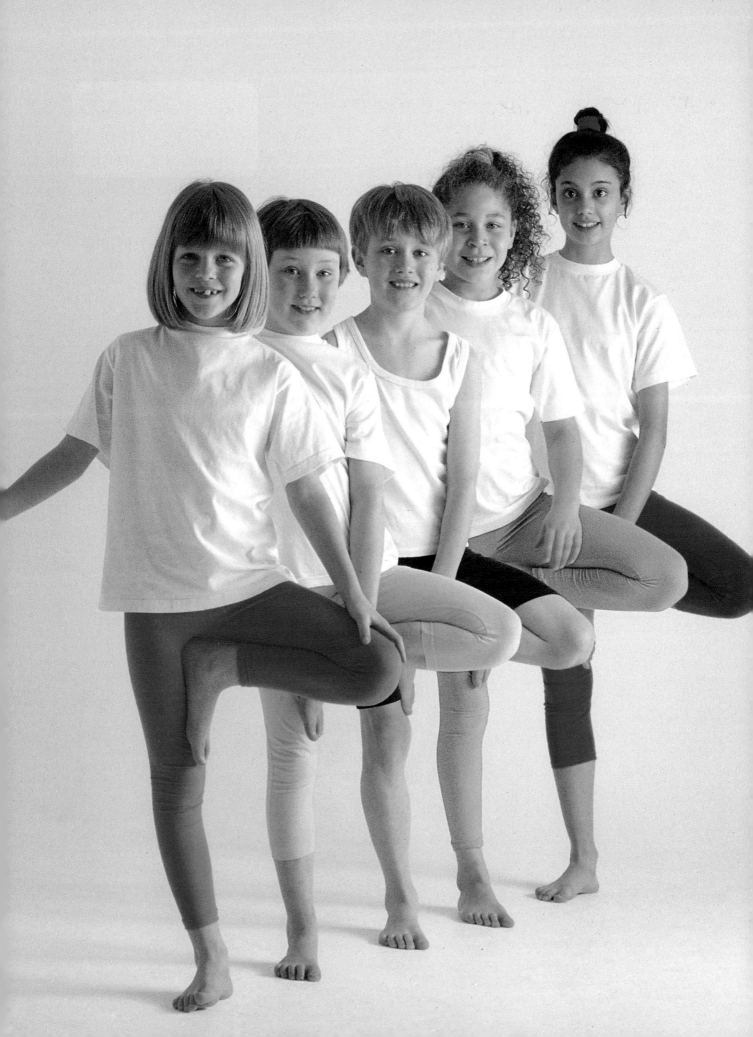

YOGA
FOR
CHILDREN

Mary Stewart and Kathy Phillips

Photography by Sandra Lousada

A Fireside Book
Published by Simon & Schuster Inc.

A Fireside Book
Published by Simon & Schuster Inc.
Simon & Schuster Building
Rockefeller Center
1230 Avenue of the Americas
New York, New York10020

10 9 8 7 6 5

Library of Congress Cataloging in Publication Data
available on request.

ISBN 0-671-78712-8

*The exercises in this book are gentle and safe
provided the instructions are followed carefully.
However, the publishers and authors disclaim all
liability in connection with the use of the information
in individual cases. If you have any doubts as to the
suitability of the exercises, consult a doctor.*

Created and designed by
Websters International Publishers Ltd, Axe and Bottle Court,
70 Newcomen Street, London SE1 1YT

CONTENTS

FIRST STEPS IN YOGA

Physical activity is natural to children and vital for their healthy development; but in today's mechanized modern society we lead much more sedentary lives than did our parents and grandparents. It is becoming difficult for some children to get the exercise they need in a natural, healthy and enjoyable way.

Yoga works on the whole body and is suitable for children of all ages and physical abilities. It promotes strength and flexibility, good coordination and posture. In our increasingly stressful and noisy lives, it teaches children how to relax, how to concentrate, how to be quiet and still. Above all, it is a gentle, noncompetitive form of exercise that all children can enjoy.

Yoga can be practiced by children in a class from the age of six. But even tiny children from three upwards can enjoy simple poses with their family.

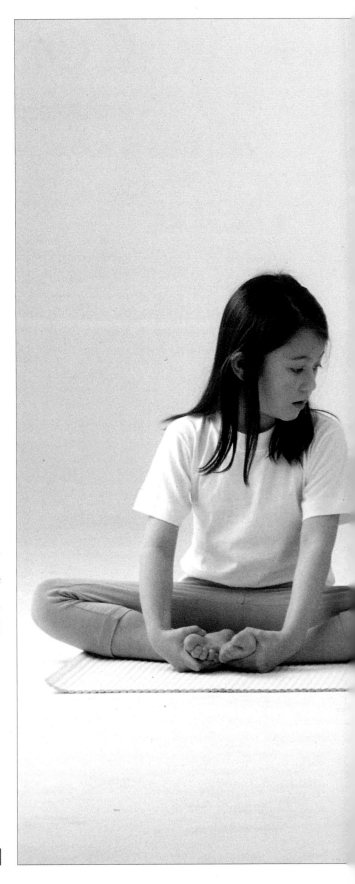

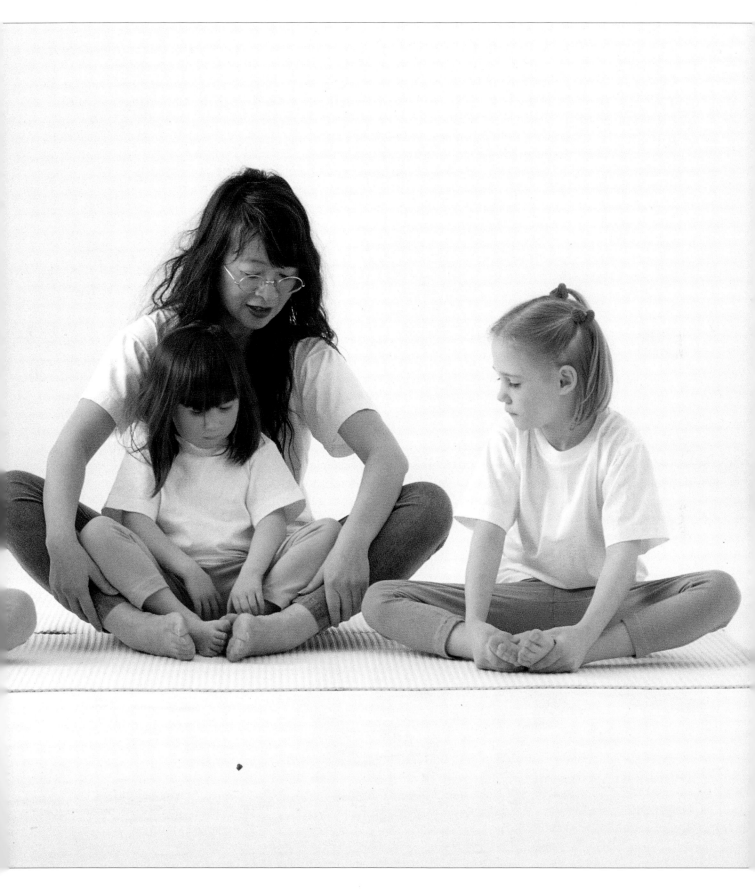

Bodies are meant to move. We need to move simply in order to stay healthy; for our joints to function properly; for our circulation to flow and our digestion to work efficiently. This applies to children every bit as much as it does to adults. Yet children nowadays - especially urban Western children - are much less active than they used to be. They spend a great deal of time sitting still in front of the television or the computer screen, and are driven everywhere by car or bus, rather than walking as they once would have done.

COMMON SENSE OF THE BODY

Children need exercise, but few people realize that the wrong kind of exercise can be as damaging as no exercise at all. Too often children are encouraged to take up vigorous and competitive exercise at a young age, unaware of the long-term problems it may cause.

When children are still growing, their bones are soft and vulnerable. Some forms of dance and gymnastics which work a young body hard can result in hip and spine problems later, not to mention arthritis. Running may well be wonderful exercise, but running with collapsed arches or hunched shoulders can do more harm than good in the long term.

In today's health-conscious world there is no shortage of advice on keeping in shape. But among all the health hype, real physical education or the teaching of a general knowledge of the body is a rare thing.

Few people of any age have the slightest idea about posture or the mechanics of their own bodies. It is as if the human biology once learned at school was not about our own bodies at all but about the structure of a remote species for which we bear no responsibility. We seem to have opted out of responsibility for our physical selves.

The result? Imbalance and instability. We spend carelessly the only capital we were born with, not noticing that our spines are becoming distorted from their natural balance or that unsuitable shoes are ruining our feet.

Physical education and sports at school are geared towards competition and performance. The 'character-building' part of such endeavors is all too often considered to be more important than simply learning how to keep the body fit for life.

Children are pushed often beyond their natural limits. Look, on the one hand, at how Olympic performers are burned out in their youth, and, on the other, at the misery of some less gifted children forced to participate in team games.

WHAT IS YOGA?

The word yoga means 'union' - a joining of the physical, mental and spiritual elements of life. Yoga poses - or asanas as they are called in Sanskrit - were developed in India centuries ago as part of a system of religious philosophy.

Yoga practice included long periods of meditation, for which you needed a trained mind and a strong body. But the poses can be employed as a straightforward form of exercise, not connected with mysticism or esoteric religions.

Yoga poses are not just physical stretches. Performed correctly with breathing, they also tone the internal organs, stimulating the body to function efficiently. The balance of quiet and active poses promotes a stability and serenity that can be useful for ordinary children, not just those who live in an ashram.

The poses in this book have been adapted to suit the life patterns of Western children. These exercises have certain advantages over other forms, especially for children: they are gentle, they are

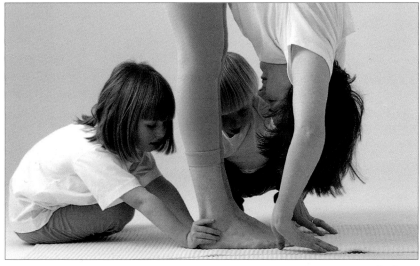

Parents who practice yoga regularly will often find that their children also become interested, and eventually they will want to join in the exercises.

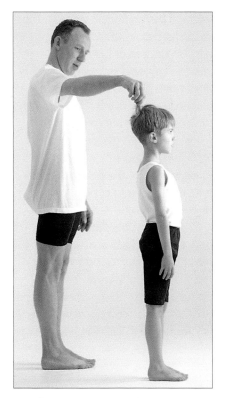

Standing up straight and tall is the basis of all yoga positions.

not performance-orientated, and they are not competitive. They can be practiced together by children of varying ages and physical abilities without anyone feeling inferior or inadequate. Yoga is not about attaining perfect poses. It is about doing what is right for your body. Every child can succeed because every child can improve.

Yoga has now become a mainstream activity for adults in the West, and it is one of the few forms of exercise that parents and children can enjoy together. They can all learn at the same time and profit equally from the experience.

WHAT YOGA DOES FOR YOU
The stretch and relaxation techniques which are part of yoga can be an ideal way for children to start enjoying movement and exercise. They can be of benefit to

children of all ages, from children as young as five or six who have already lost the flexibility they had as babies to teenagers contending with pressures of school and the emotional problems of adolescence.

Yoga exercises are not ends in themselves. They do certain very specific things not just for your body but for your whole sense of mental and physical well-being. They enhance your flexibility; they promote your strength and stamina, stability and balance; they help you to relax but at the same time to become more concentrated, more clear-headed, less distracted; to become alert while being tranquil.

Not forcing yourself further than is realistic is an important lesson. Yoga will help children learn about the body and how it works from a very early age. It will help them develop that common sense of the body which is the perfect foundation for their well-being throughout their lives.

WORK
In the chapters entitled 'Work' poses have been chosen to move, bend and stretch the body. Each part of the body is tackled. Learning how to stand and stretch, using the pull of gravity, helps with balance and concentration. All the joints will become strong and flexible. These poses are grouped into standing poses, all-fours poses, balancing poses, sitting poses, upside down poses and back bends.

REST
This section concentrates on the need for quiet. As the body gets tense so does the mind,

particularly a child's mind over-stimulated by the pace of life, television, computer games and noise. By learning to breathe deeply, and to lie and sit still without wiggling about, they are given the chance to appreciate time and space to be silent.

PLAY
This section offers games for children to enjoy in a group as well as for parents to play with their children. They have been devised using the poses explained in the previous chapters and encourage coordination and teamwork. They also allow children to jump, run and generally let off steam.

NEEDS
Yoga is particularly helpful for those with special needs, whether they are the result of bad posture or sporting practices leading to tension and stiffness, or whether

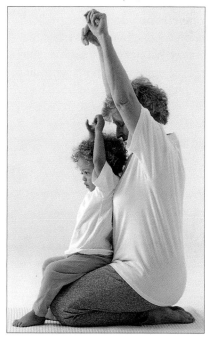

Even very small children like getting involved in yoga sessions.

9

they stem from a more serious disability. This section includes advice for correcting stiffness as well as simple poses to benefit disabled children. In some cases it is amazing to discover that the disabled child is more flexible than the so-called able-bodied. Sometimes, too, a disabled child can find it easier to be quiet and centered. The shared Yoga class is an occasion for everybody to learn from one another.

PRACTICING YOGA

Because children have a short concentration span, time spent learning yoga must be fun. As a start, the positions in this book have been given special names which may not always be exact translations from the Sanskrit (though the actual Sanskrit is also given for those who are interested), but they sound as if they promise enjoyment and children will find them more approachable.

It is important to be properly prepared for yoga. Wear comfortable clothes, ones that are stretchy but not tight - such as the T-shirts, tights and shorts worn in our pictures. Practice in bare feet on a non-slip surface such as a wooden or cork-tiled floor, or certain types of carpet. If the room is really cold, have a warm sweater and socks ready to put on when resting at the end of the session.

No special equipment is needed for yoga though certain props may come in useful. A stool or chair is helpful for some people in some poses (see page 29) and a belt in

All yoga sessions should end with Dead Man's Pose - lying straight and completely flat on the floor.

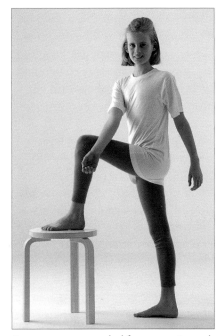

Few props are needed for yoga. A stool is helpful in some positions.

others (page 70). For some of the upside-down poses, and some sitting poses you will need a mat or folded blanket.

BASIC PRINCIPLES

When they are learning yoga all children should be supervised until they understand what they are doing. Working in a group with a parent or adult is the best way to learn the basic principles. Eventually older children should be able to follow the instructions for themselves.

Look at the photographs and

read the instructions carefully. The positions should not be held for too long - a couple of breaths for small children; older children can stay a little longer provided they continue to stretch comfortably. You should not freeze in an uncomfortable position. It is not an endurance test. Hold poses for an equal time on each side of the body. Breathe out as you go into a pose, otherwise breathe naturally.

A yoga session should last as long as everybody is enjoying it - but at most for about 45 minutes, and the last ten minutes of that should be spent doing something quiet. Adults usually practice every day, but once a week is fine for children. A teenager under study stress, however, would also benefit from practicing every day, if only for ten minutes.

The poses in this book have been carefully chosen to be safe and suitable for children. But it is important to follow the instructions and not to allow children to push themselves too far. If in doubt consult a doctor. In some yoga books you will find other, more advanced poses and these should not be attempted by children. Headstands and extreme back bends are inadvisable as children's bones are still soft and the neck is vulnerable. Don't forget that rest should always follow work poses.

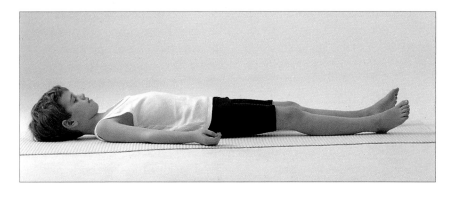

THE BASIC PROGRAM

It is important to practice the yoga poses in sequence. Each program should include poses that stretch the body into action and provide a balance of quiet and relaxation. The sequence is not a rigid ritual that you have to stick to like glue. You can choose the poses you do as long as you follow certain general principles:

Warm-up - Start off with something that earths you to the floor. This can be a standing pose, the gravity game or shoulder flopping. Feel that you're completely grounded and straight before going on to the next stage. However, if you have a specific problem with stiffness, this is the point to practice something from the Needs section.

Action - Now for the more challenging poses. All these appear in the 'Work' section. Choose a variety of poses from the different parts of the section, so that you stretch your body in different ways - forwards, backwards and twisting.

Game - This is for children working in a group to let off steam and have fun before becoming quiet. Choose a game which uses poses previously learned.

Winding down - It will take a little time to quiet down. If you have stretched the body hard in one direction, choose a quiet pose that stretches it the other way.

Being quiet - Be silent for a few minutes, either sitting or lying.

Lying flat - Always end with Dead Man's Pose (page 96). This experience of total quiet is the cornerstone of yoga practice.

The suggestions for programs

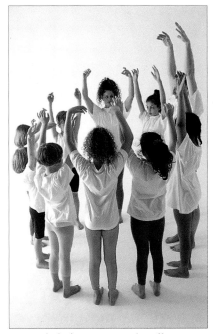

Games help large groups let off steam before quieting down.

that follow give you some examples of how these principles might work out in practice. Then make up your own.

PROGRAMS:	ONE	TWO	THREE	FOUR
Warm-up	Gravity Game Tree Triangle	Mountain Warrior Rag Doll	Mountain	Mountain Triangle Standing Twist
Action	Cat Bird Plow Butterfly	Dog Snake Candle	Sundance	Scissors Locust Sandwich
Game	Mother's trees	Bowling	Sunwheel	Crocodile
Winding down	Buzzing	Bell Game	Snooze	Snooze
Being quiet	Lying flat arms wrapped	Finding your breath	Diamond	Lying flat knees bent up
Lying flat	Dead Man's Pose	Dead Man's Pose	Dead Man's Pose	Dead Man's Pose

WORK

Yoga poses tone and straighten the body keeping it strong and flexible. The work poses are the active ones - positions that stretch the spine from a stable and rooted base, whether standing or sitting, balancing, on all fours, or upside down.

The work poses help the body grow straight, free and balanced. Each pose is a gentle movement, and you should use your breath like a wave carrying you along to stretch further. Breathing out as you go into a pose helps the spine to lengthen. This way your body is never forced, or pushed to extremes.

The Wheel is an advanced yoga pose that makes you super-flexible and gives you energy. Done correctly, the spine lengthens and the lower back is free.

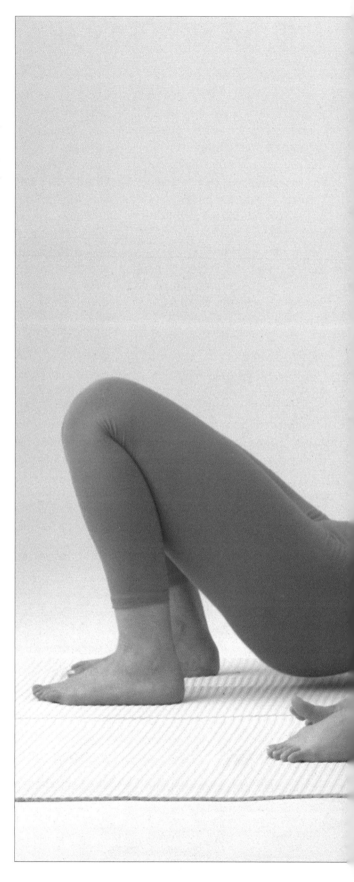

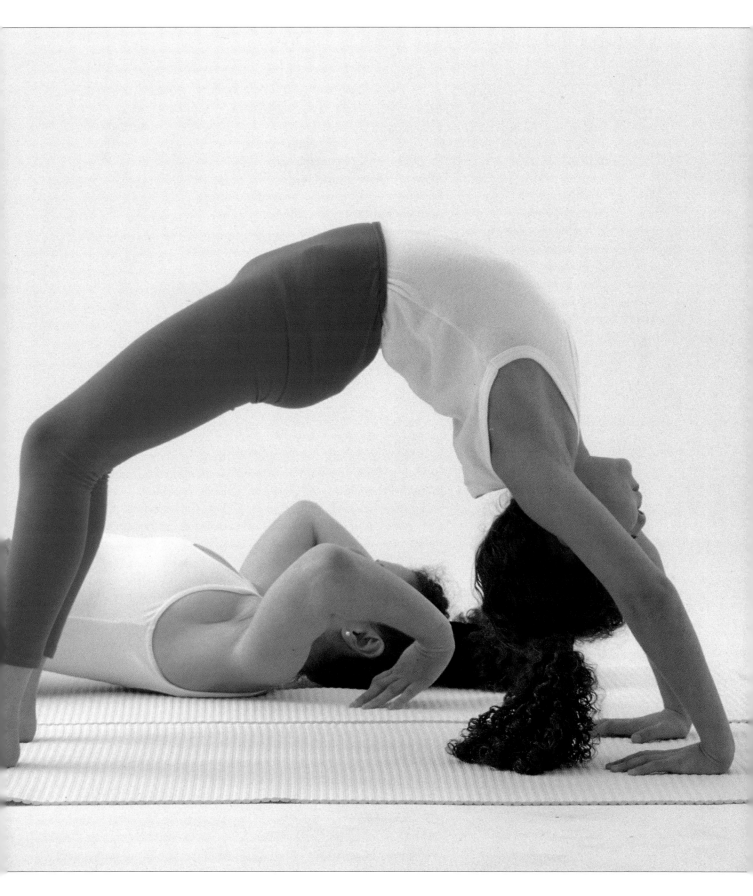

Your body is a connected whole. Each bit affects the next. Remember the song about your kneebone being connected to your thighbone, your thighbone to your hipbone, and so on? All the parts of the body must move easily in order for the body to function to its full potential. The work poses are the ones which stretch all these different parts. They grow organically from a rooted base so that the spine becomes taller. This is true whether the pose is a standing pose, or on all fours, balancing, sitting, upside down or a back bend. When they are functioning well the parts of the body move in different ways.

SPINE

The spine is the structural center of the body and it should be looked after from childhood on. It should never be squashed or distorted or compressed. It balances in four curves - at the neck, the chest, the

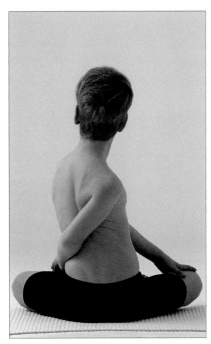

Your spine should be able to twist while staying straight and upright.

waist and the hips - and is made up of a string of small bones, separated by discs of cartilage. This is what makes the spine so flexible, but it is this very flexibility that makes it possible for bad habits to distort it. A healthy spine should be able to lengthen and move in different directions - forwards, backwards, sideways and twisting - while keeping straight at the same time.

FEET

Feet are the root of all our standing movements - the foundation of every pose. How your feet work affects how you walk, run, stand and balance. How your feet carry your weight ultimately affects the action of your knees, hips and ankles

Feet are shock absorbers as well as being the foundation of all standing movements. Feet should be strong, firm, flexible and arched. When you stand put your weight on your heels so that you can spread your toes out wide and the arches of your feet can be strong and springy. Standing correctly grounded will allow the rest of your body to relax and stay free.

SHOULDERS

Shoulders are the most mobile joints in the body. As long as they are relaxed the arms can move freely in all directions. If shoulders are moving properly you should easily be able to hold both elbows behind your back, and stretch your arms straight above your head.

HIPS

The hips are ball and socket joints and should have a wide range of movement. They are also weight-

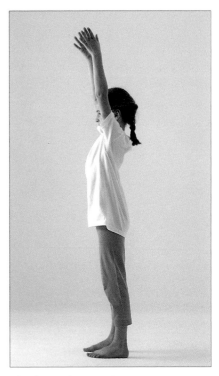

The force of gravity helps you stand tall from a firm base.

bearing joints and must be working symmetrically if the whole body is not to be thrown out of line. Sitting poses and upside down poses help to develop mobility.

LEGS AND KNEES

The main movement in the legs comes from the hips. Everyone should be able to touch their toes by bending forward from the hips with knees straight. Tight hamstrings can prevent this and cause strain on the lower back.

Knees are hinge joints and should be able to bend fully and straighten.

GRAVITY

Gravity is an important factor in all movement. You need to understand how the body is grounded to the earth. If you stand really centered you will feel how your body spontaneously grows taller. In contrast, continual bad posture can take you out of alignment.

BREATHING
Learning to breathe is as important as understanding how your body moves. The breath, which comes from your center, helps you to stretch and elongate. Always breathe out as you go into a pose.

THE POSES
The work poses are divided into six groups: standing, all fours, balancing, sitting, upside down and back bends. Each position needs firm roots so that you can stretch evenly and grow tall and straight. The roots of a standing pose are the feet, those of a sitting pose the sitting bones, those of a balancing pose the hands, those of inverted poses the elbows. In each case, the roots of the position go down into the ground so that the spine stretches as you breathe out. Each practice session should contain poses from several of these groups, and work poses should be followed by rest.

Standing In these poses the feet are the roots of the pose, and the spine lengthens as you stand and

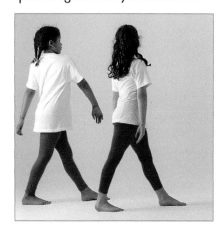

The feet, with the weight on the heels, are the roots of all standing poses.

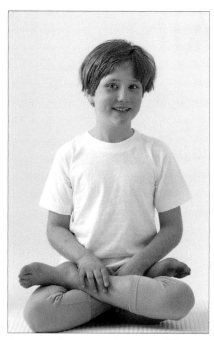

The sitting bones are the roots of the sitting poses, such as Lotus (page 88).

walk and balance. Learning to be grounded as well as relaxed when you are a child is more valuable than having to correct bad posture by learning a technique when you are older.

All fours Some of the Yoga poses copy the movements of animals. Many postural problems arise because you balance badly on two feet and the spine does not have a chance to stretch. Here on all fours you can lengthen like a cat or dog and iron out the bends and stiffnesses in your spine.

Balancing These are poses where you shift the weight on to your hands in order to balance. Children develop coordination and strength from these exercises although they are not suitable for the under fives.

Sitting It is vital to learn how to sit properly with flexible hips and the spine long and free. Sitting poses work mainly on the hips. Their roots are the two sitting bones - the

knobbly bones under the pelvis. If the floor is hard you may need a mat or blanket for these poses.

Upside down Turning upside down reverses the pull of gravity and is a wonderful way of stretching. Upside down you can stretch legs and hips more easily because they are not bearing any weight. These poses are also a way of keeping the upper spine and neck flexible. When you are practicing them always lengthen your neck with your shoulders as you go up. You should not compress the neck in upside down poses.

Back bends Back bends are invigorating, and will also keep you flexible. But doing this movement badly causes more problems than with any other pose. The danger is that, in an effort to bend, you may forget to lengthen the spine. This can compress the back of the waist and neck and cause stiffness and distortion of the spine later. It is also important to use a nonslip mat for these poses if the floor is slippery. Pay attention to the instructions and be sure to keep your heels down and feet parallel when doing Wheel. This way the spine can lengthen and the lower back is free.

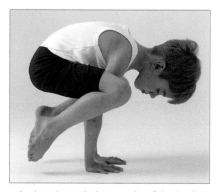

The hands, with the weight of the body on the heels of the hands, are the roots of balancing poses, such as Bird (page 36).

MOUNTAIN

Tadasana

A mountain rises out of the earth, its peak high up in the clouds. In this pose plant your feet into the ground beneath and grow tall until your head touches the sky. This is the start of all the standing poses.

Stand with your feet slightly apart and parallel. Keep your legs straight, weight on your heels, and toes spread out. You are anchored to the floor by your legs and heels, which allows your spine to straighten as you stretch up.

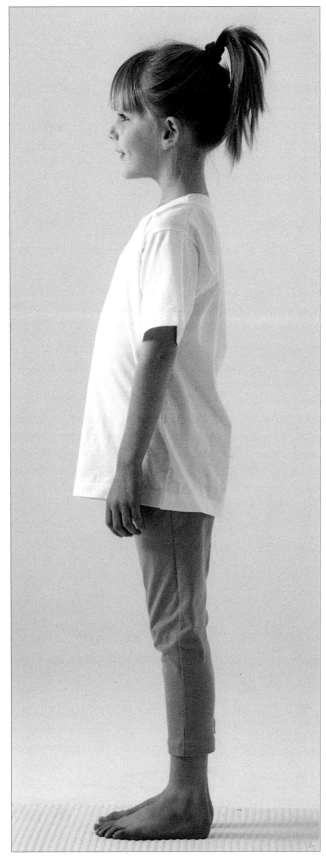

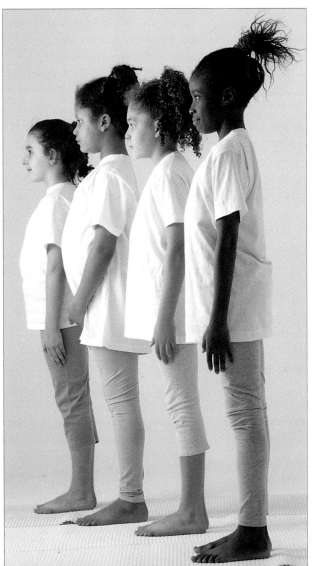

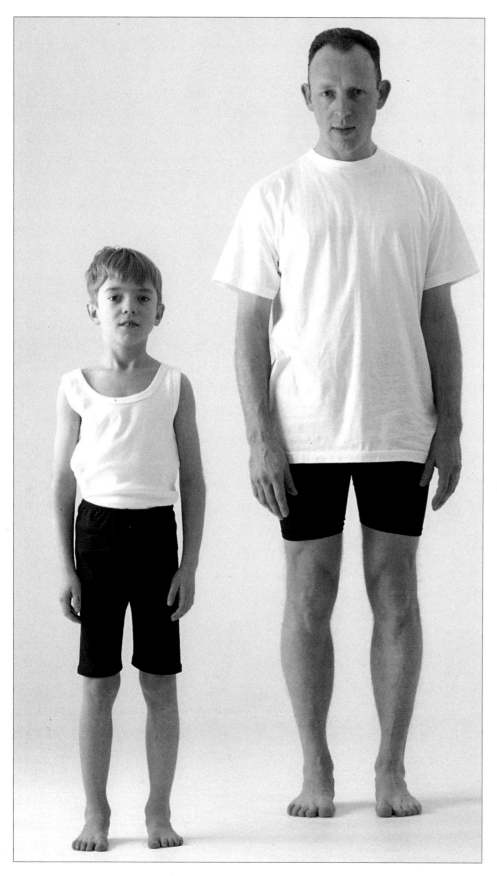

Be sure that you are standing evenly on both feet and let your arms and shoulders relax. This pose should be stable without being stiff or rigid. Let your head balance naturally on top of your spine.

TREE

Vrksasana

A tree will only grow tall if its roots go deep down into the earth. Your standing leg is the root of the tree, your spine is the trunk, your arms the branches.

1 Stand up straight as in Mountain pose. Keep your shoulders relaxed and down, the back of your neck long, and your chin slightly tucked in.

2 Keep your left leg straight. Breathe out, take your right foot and place it high on the inside of your left thigh.

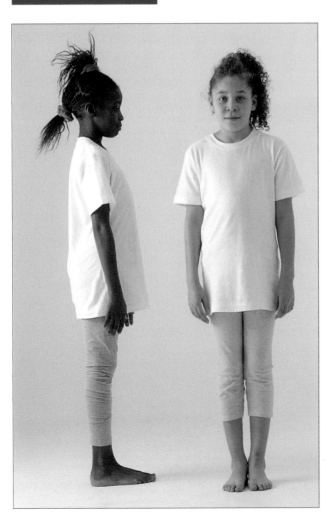

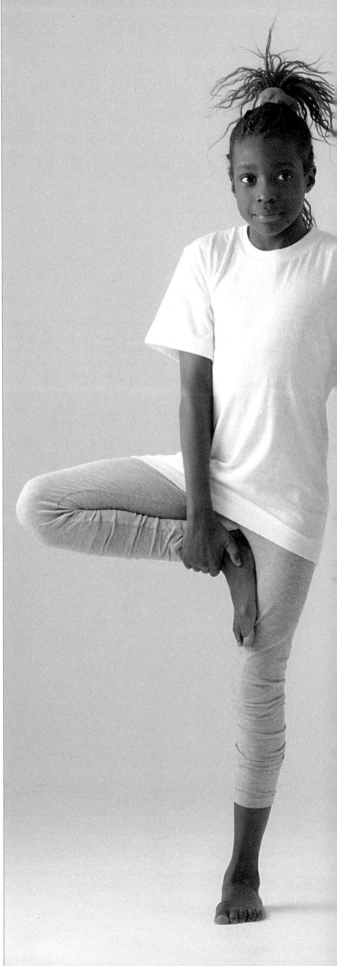

18

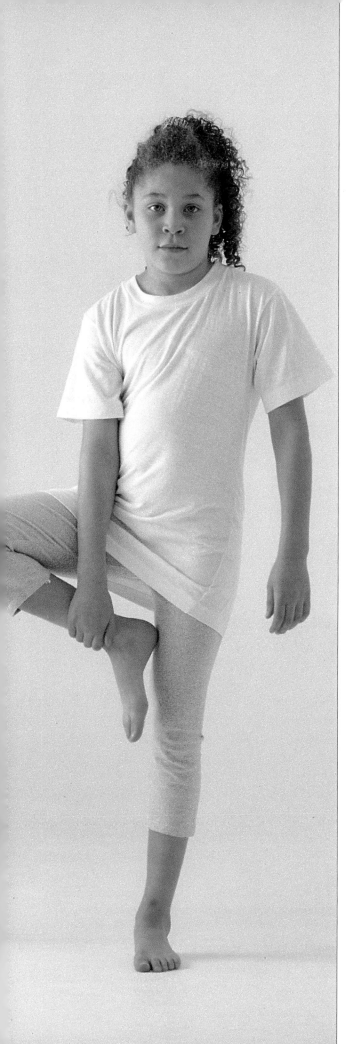

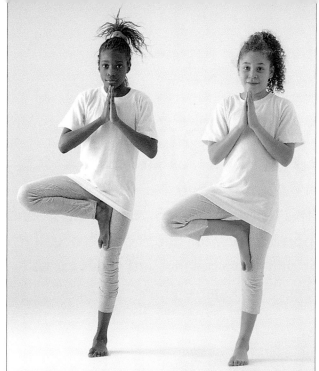

3 Your weight should be on the heel of the standing foot which goes down into the ground like a tree root. Relax your shoulders and put the palms of your hands together.

4 Slowly raise your arms above your head like tree branches. Come down and repeat the pose standing on your right leg and raising your left foot.

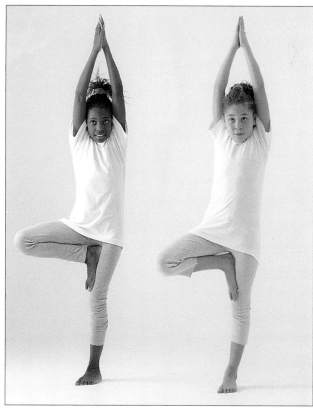

WARRIOR

Virabhadrasana

This warrior is strong, steady, alert - and poised ready for attack or defence. If it is difficult to balance just go as far as step 3 to begin with.

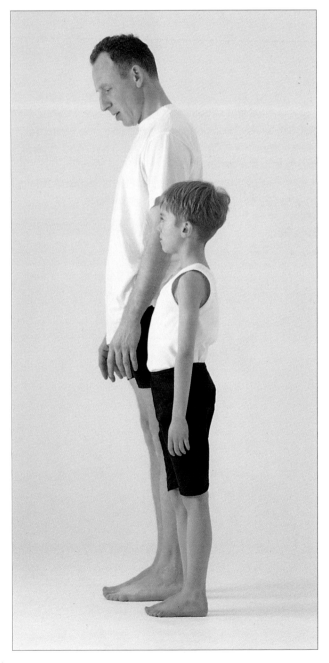

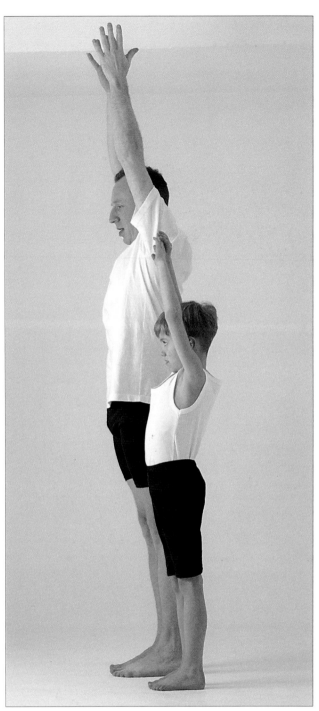

1 Stand tall as in Mountain pose, feet pointing forward, slightly apart and parallel.

2 Breathe out and lift both arms straight up above your head. Don't tighten your shoulders.

20

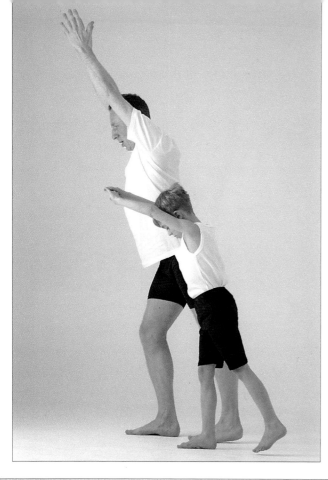

3 Place your right foot one step forwards, keeping the weight on the back heel. Grow tall from the back heel to your fingertips. Let the right leg bend. Breathe out and stretch upwards and forwards, transferring your weight on to your right foot. Your left foot will come off the floor. Keep the left leg straight, knee facing the floor.

4 Your back leg carries on stretching away from you as it swings up. Straighten your right leg and balance, lengthening your spine as the heel of the raised foot stretches away. Come back to the original position and repeat the pose on the left leg.

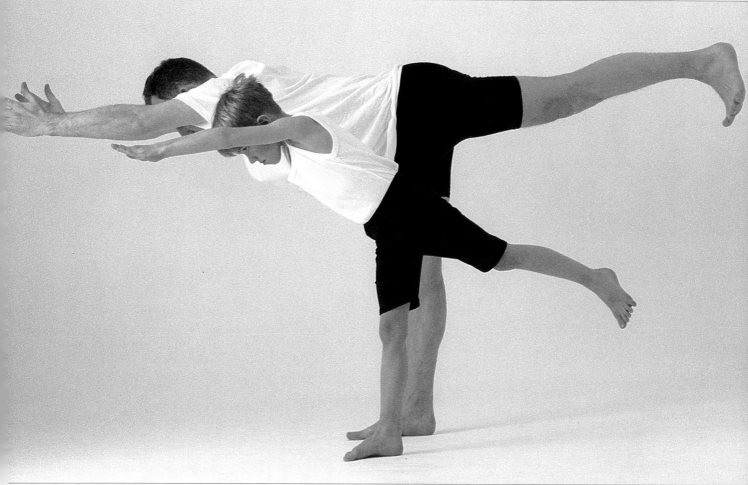

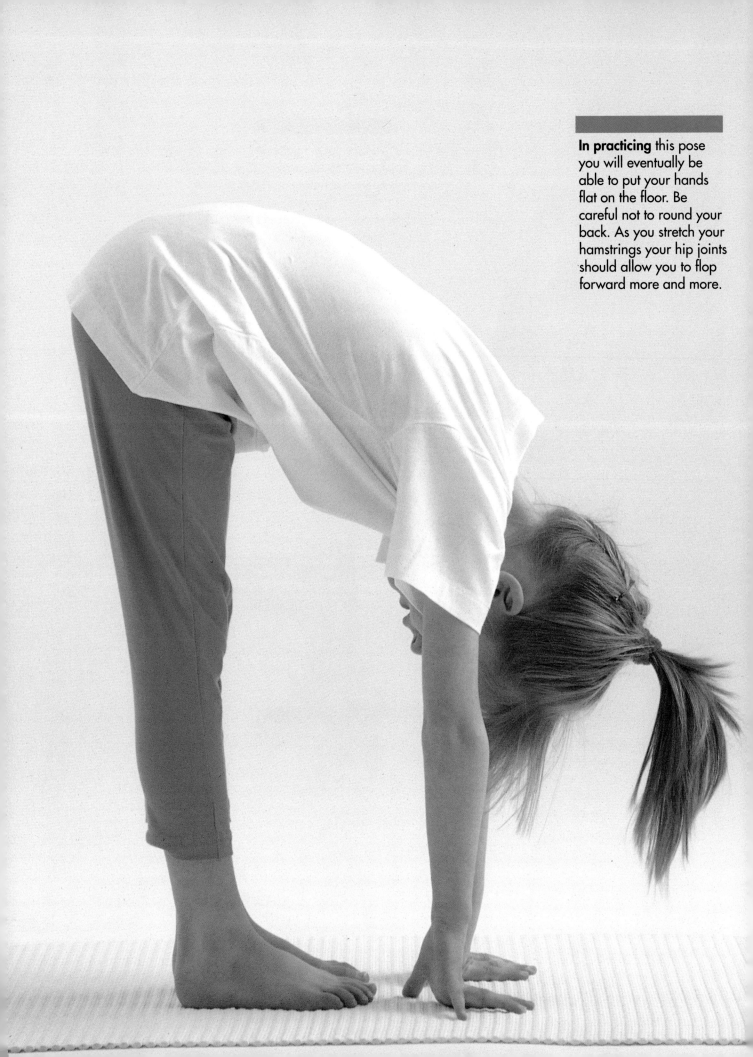

In practicing this pose you will eventually be able to put your hands flat on the floor. Be careful not to round your back. As you stretch your hamstrings your hip joints should allow you to flop forward more and more.

RAG DOLL

Uttanasana

In this pose you are like a doll that bends in the middle and flops forward. Your legs stay straight and firm, your body hangs down and your arms fall towards the floor.

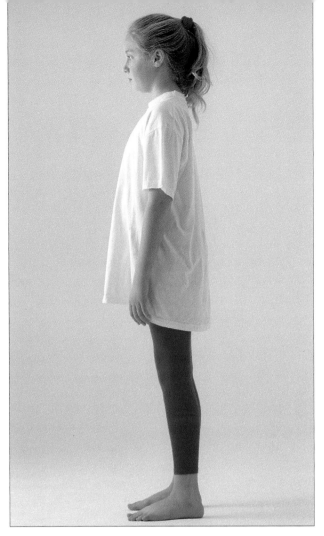

1 Stand straight and tall as in Mountain pose with your shoulders down, head straight and the back of your neck long.

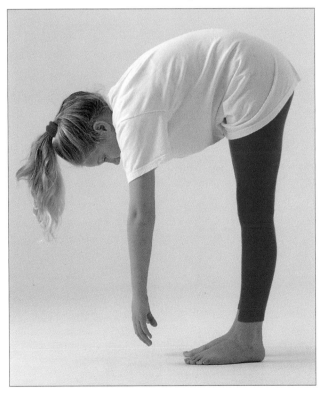

If the backs of your legs are stiff and you can't lengthen your back as you go forwards to touch the floor, put your hands on a stool or chair.

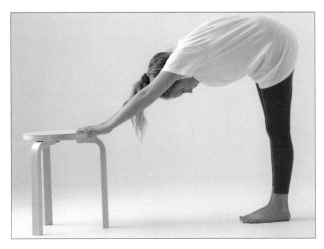

2 With your heels down and the back of your knees straight, breathe out and bend from the hips so that your arms flop down. Keep your weight even on both feet. Breathe out as you come up.

23

TRIANGLE

Trikonasana

The base of the pose is the triangle made by your legs and the floor. Keep your knees straight so that the triangle stays strong. The pose stretches the spine sideways and loosens the shoulders.

1 Stand straight and tall as in Mountain pose.

2 Place the right foot a walking pace forwards, keeping the weight on the back foot. The toes of both feet should point forwards.

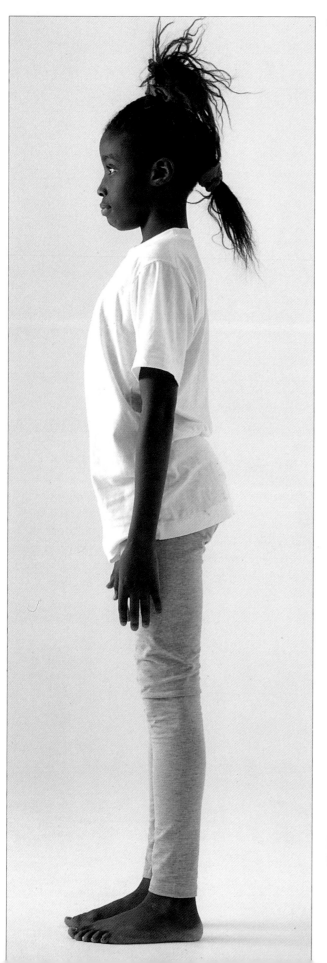

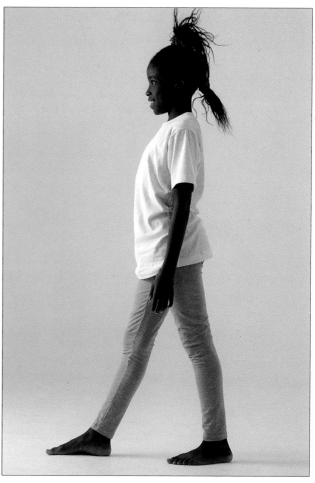

3 Keeping the weight on the back foot, and the toes still pointing forwards, turn to the left extending your left arm away from you.

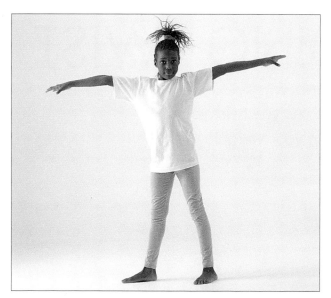

4 Breathe out and lengthen your spine to the right as you bend over sideways. Keep your shoulders relaxed. Come up gently and repeat on the other side.

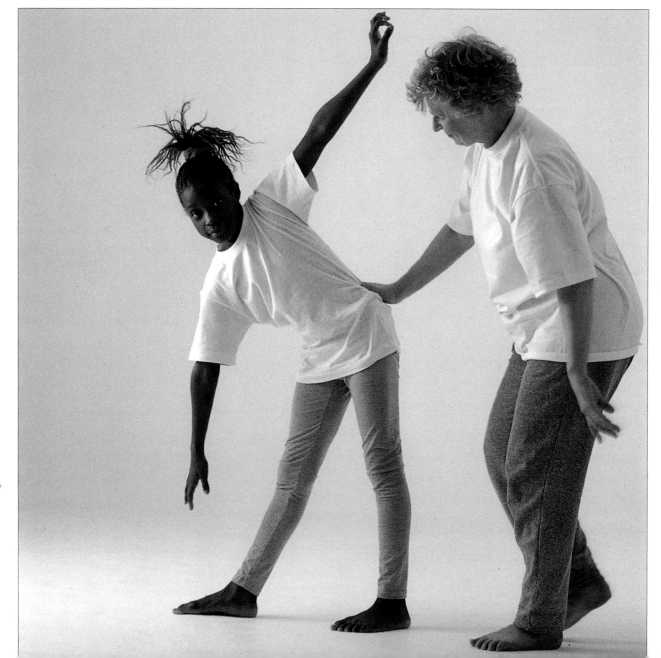

STANDING TWIST

Parivrtta Trikonasana

This is a walking pose. As you twist your
body you have to keep your weight
firmly on your back heel.

1 Stand straight and tall
as in Mountain pose.
Place your right foot one
step forwards, keeping
your weight on your back
foot, as in Triangle.

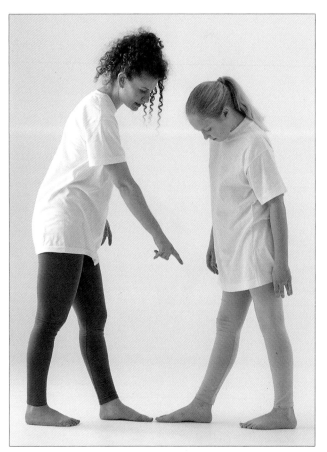

2 With your toes still
pointing forwards,
breathe out and turn to
the right extending your
arms sideways. This pose
is more difficult than
Triangle as your heel
tends to lift off the floor
as you turn.

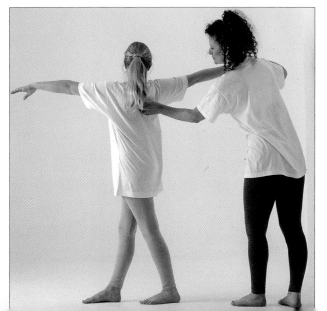

26

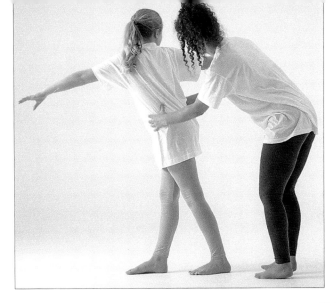

3 Turn more and look at your right hand. Keeping your left heel down and your shoulders relaxed, stretch your spine as far as you can. Breathe out as you come up. Repeat on the other side.

For your spine to lengthen in this pose, you have to be firmly anchored by your back heel with your shoulders relaxed.

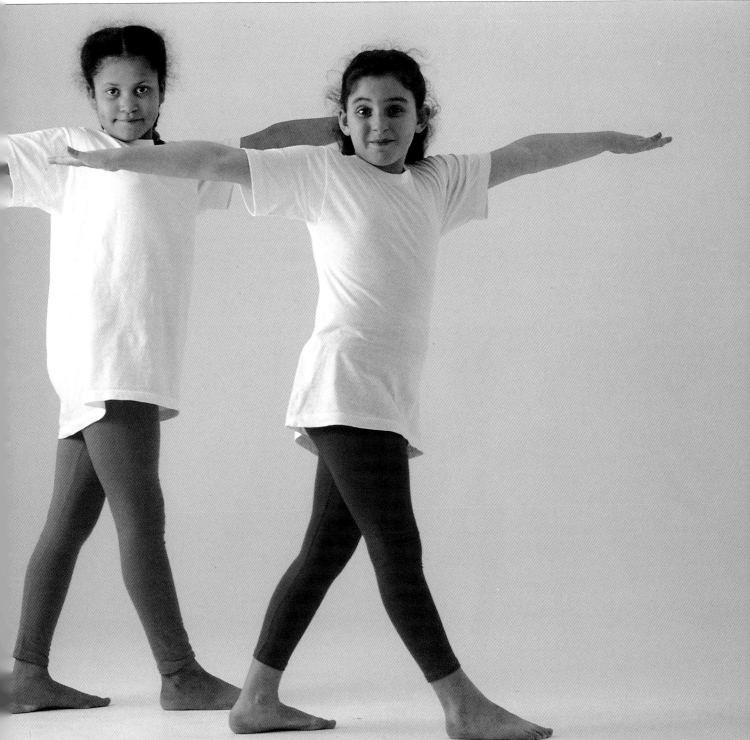

WIGWAM

Prasarita Padottanasana

In this pose your legs and body make the shape of a tent. Keep your legs and back as straight as possible. If your legs are too far apart the tent will collapse, if they are too close together there will be no room inside.

1 Stand with the legs apart, toes pointing forward and parallel.

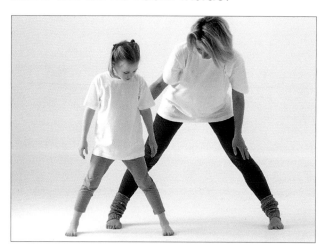

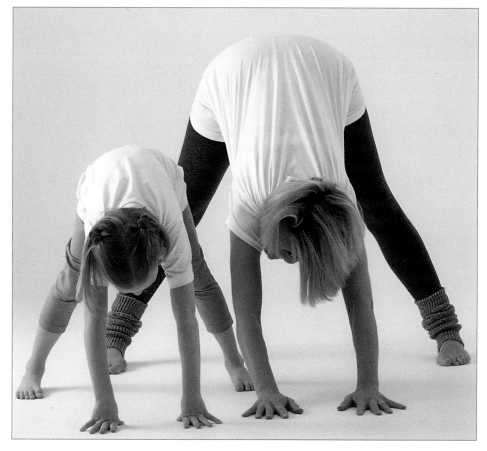

2 Breathe out, bend forward from the hips and place your hands on the floor in front of you. Keep your weight firmly on your heels and concentrate on stretching your spine forwards.

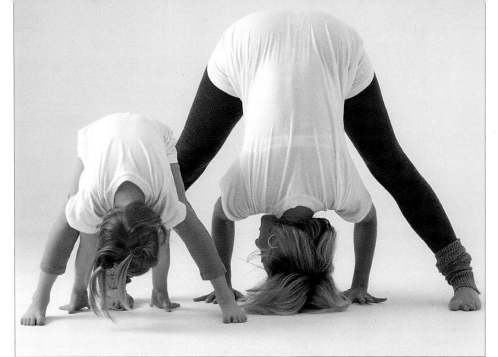

3 Bend your elbows placing your palms in line with your feet. Breathe out and lengthen your spine until your head touches the floor.

If the backs of your legs are stiff go forwards on to a stool. Breathe out and come up slowly.

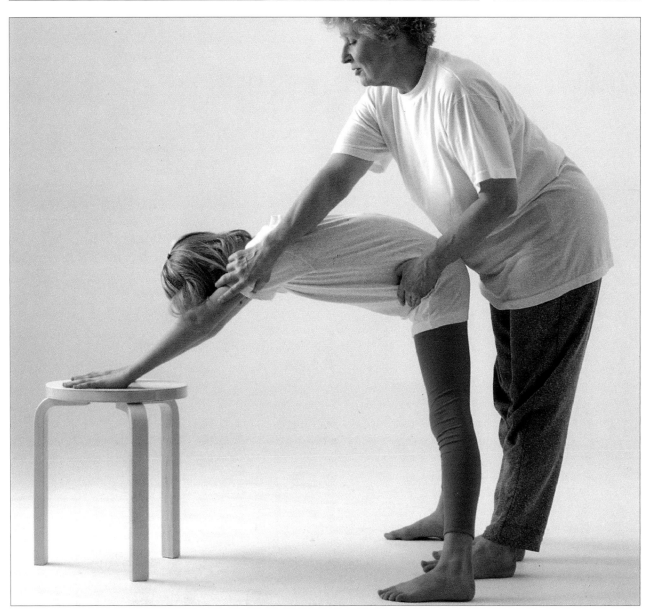

SQUAT
Malasana

Although you are squatting your feet should be as firmly rooted to the ground as in the other standing poses.

1 Stand straight and tall as in Mountain pose, with shoulders relaxed. Your weight should be on your heels.

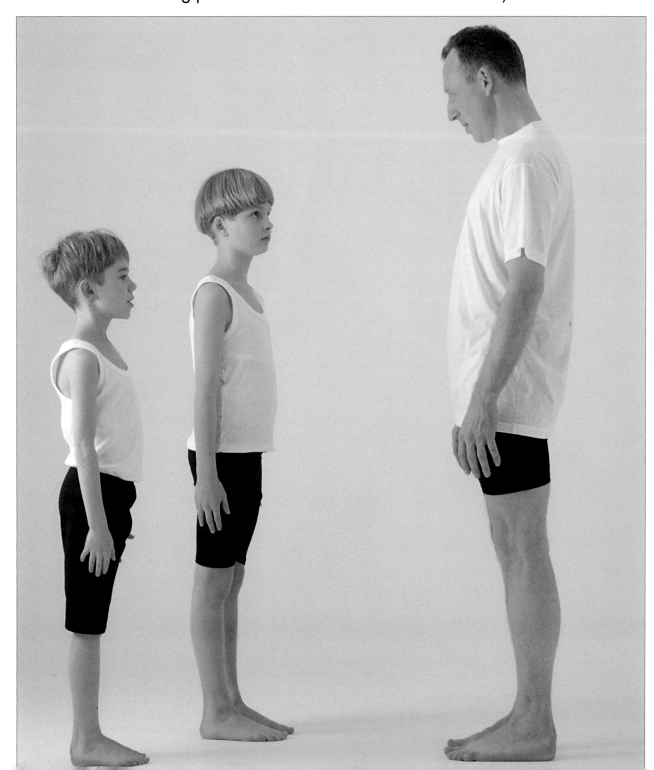

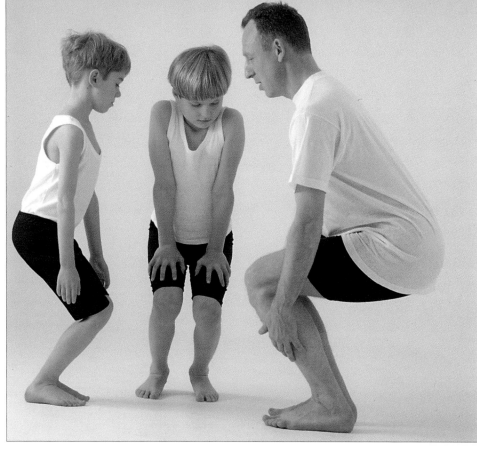

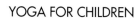

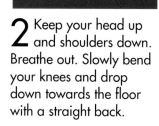

2 Keep your head up and shoulders down. Breathe out. Slowly bend your knees and drop down towards the floor with a straight back.

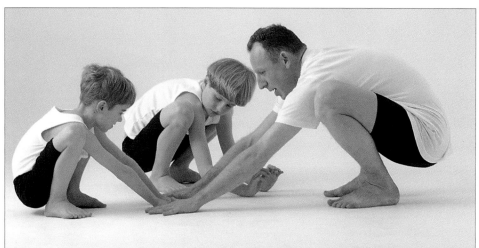

3 Balance in squatting position with heels flat on the floor and head up. Place your hands forwards on the floor in front of you.

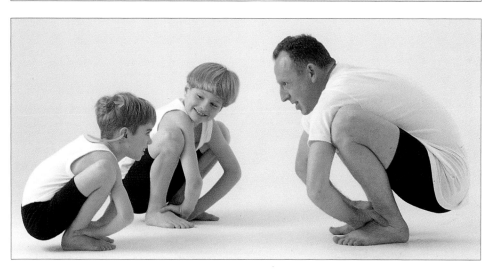

4 Breathe out again and drop your elbows down towards the floor, letting them bend so that you can turn your hands back to hold your ankles. In this finished position the Squat is known as Garland pose.

DOG

Adho Mukha Svanasana

This is how a dog gets up after a good sleep. It lifts its tail high in the air as it stretches its front paws out. The aim of the pose is to stretch out fully with straight knees and feet flat on the floor.

1 Start on all fours with the palms of your hands and your knees on the floor, arms straight.

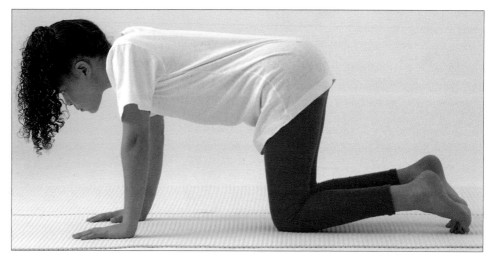

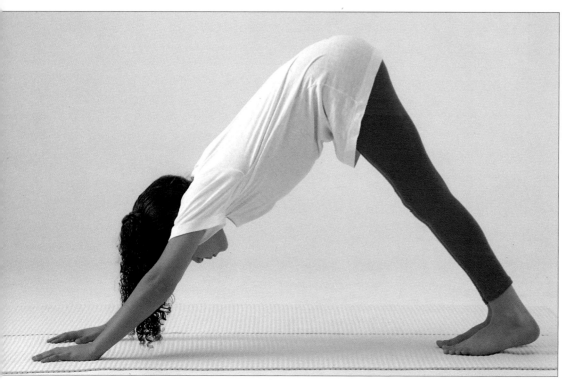

2 Breathe out. Tuck your toes under and lift up your hips and buttocks, slowly straightening your legs.

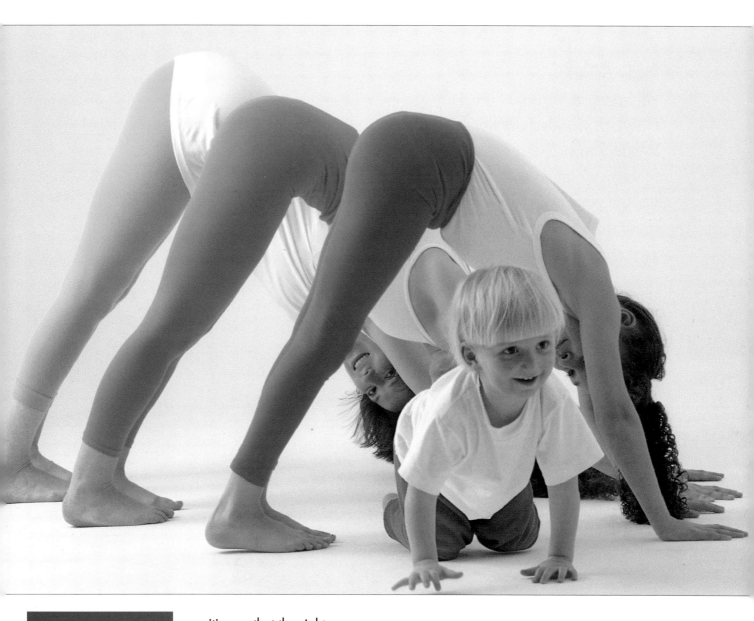

3 Now stretch more, just like like a dog, so that your arms and legs are straight, and your weight is back as far as you can make it on to your heels. Adjust your position so that the right and left sides of your body stretch evenly and you make a triangle with the floor. Bend your knees and sit gently down on your heels, bend forward and relax.

CAT

Bidalasana

Cats are wonderfully flexible animals. When you stroke a cat you can actually feel its spine move. In this pose you hollow your back, then arch it high - as a cat does when it's frightened or cross.

1 Kneel on all fours with the palms of your hands flat on the floor shoulder width apart. Your fingers should be pointing forwards and your toes back. Keep your arms straight.

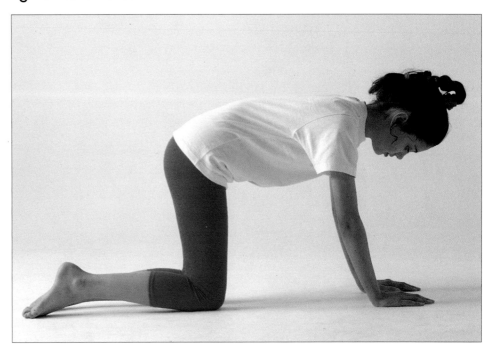

2 As you breathe out hollow your back, keeping your arms straight and your shoulders relaxed.

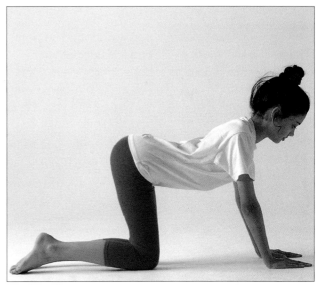

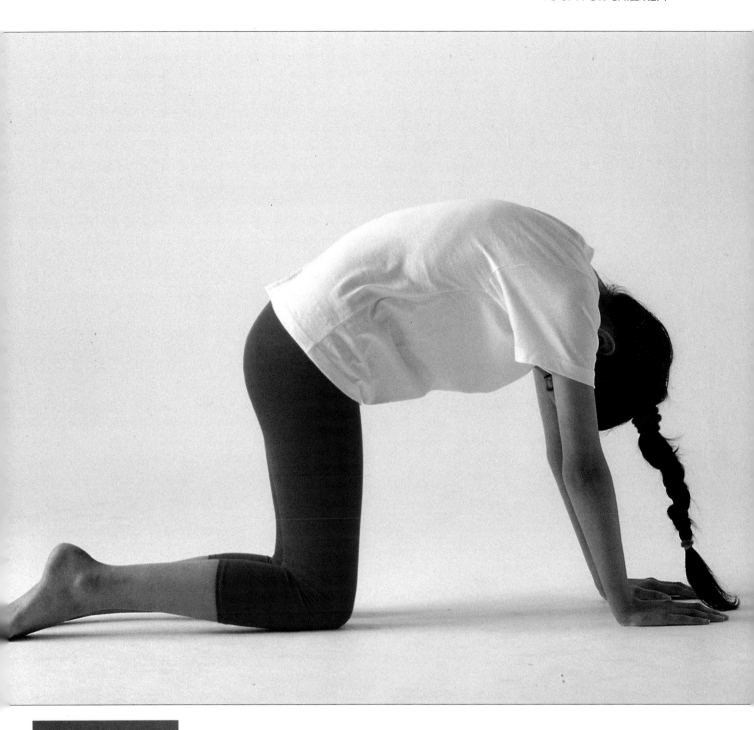

3 On the next out-breath arch your back in the opposite direction. You like you can make a hissing noise like an angry cat as you do this. Come back to the original position.

BIRD
Bakasana

A bird has long legs and a small light body. In this pose your hands are the bird's feet and your arms are its legs.

1 Start in the squatting position with parallel feet flat on the floor and your hands shoulder width apart on the floor in front of you. Your shoulders should be inside your knees.

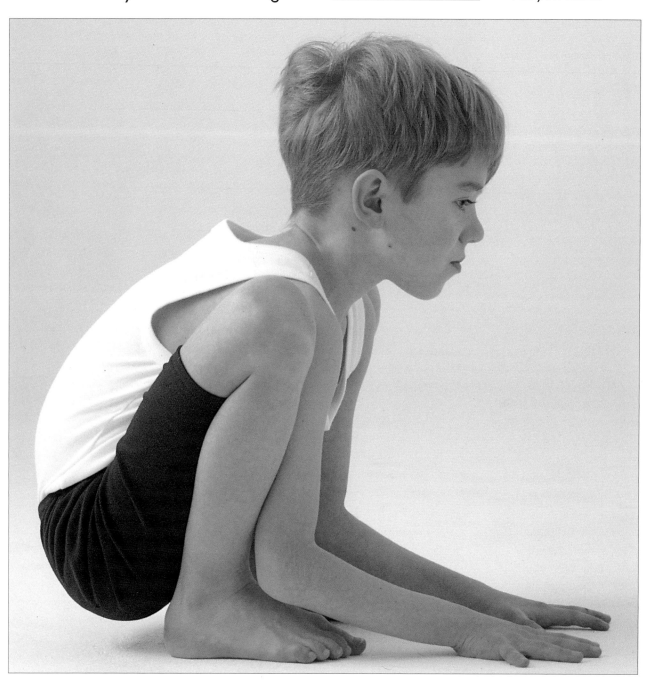

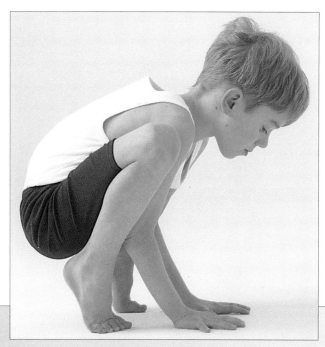

2 Breathe out, lift up on to your toes and let your weight rock forwards on to your hands. Your hands must be firmly planted on the ground as they are the roots of balancing poses. Keep your knees in and your feet as close together as you can.

3 Straighten your arms as your feet lift off the floor. Keep your head up and your neck long as you move forwards to balance on your hands.

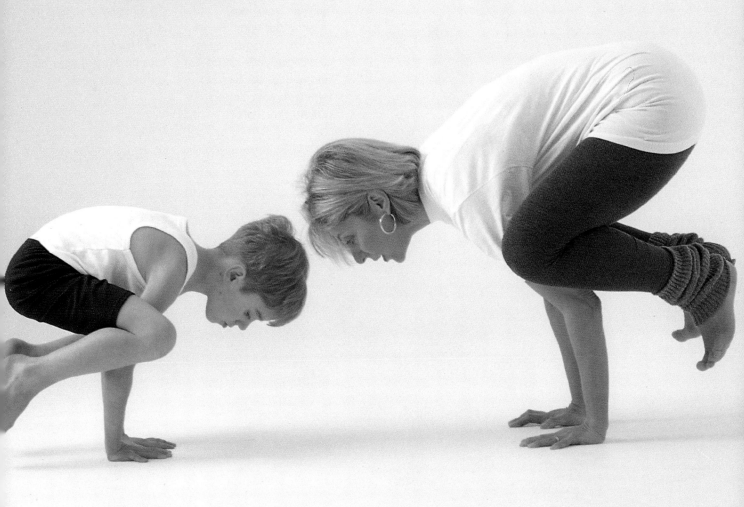

FLYING BIRD

Bhujapidasana

This is another bird pose where you balance on the heels of your hands, but this time the bird is about to spread its wings and fly away.

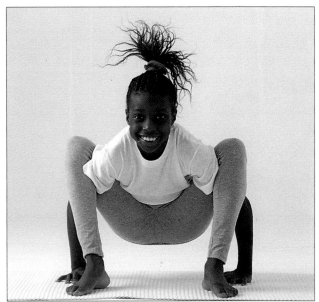

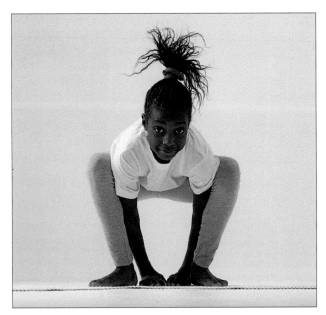

1 With your legs shoulder width apart breathe out, squat down and place your hands flat on the floor inside your feet, with your fingers pointing forwards.

2 One by one, wiggle your shoulders underneath your knees. Your hands will now be behind your heels.

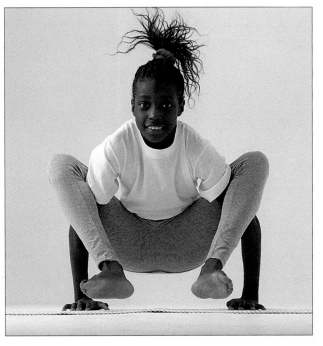

3 Breathe out and let your weight move on to your hands so that your feet begin to come off the floor. Grip in with your knees.

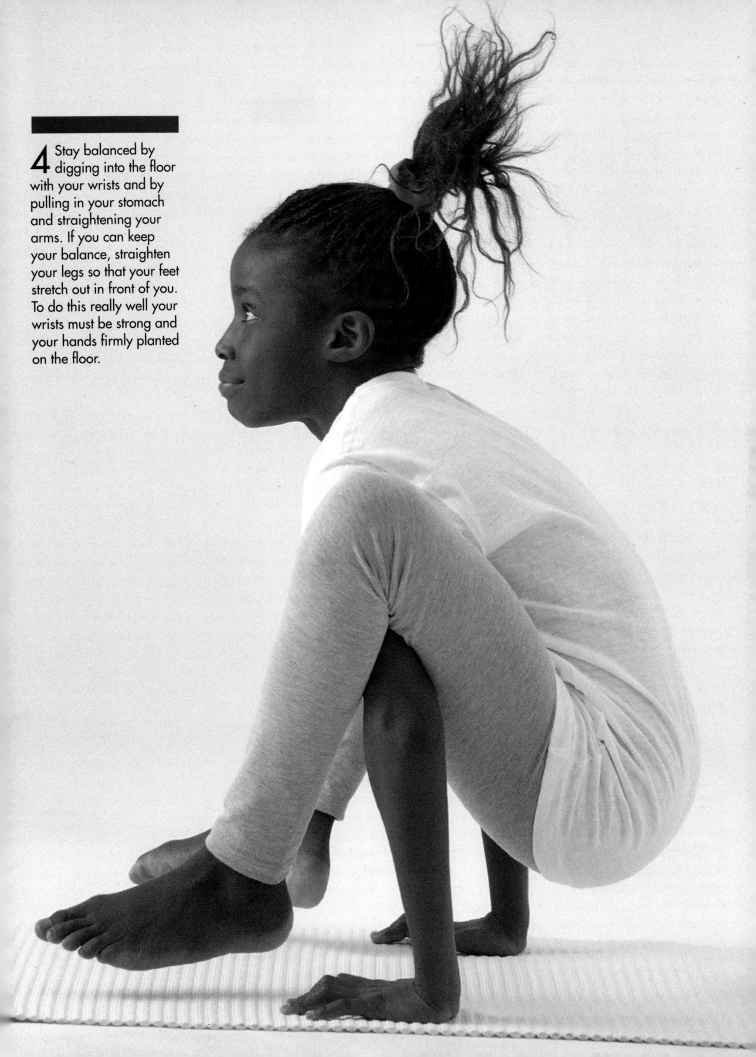

4 Stay balanced by digging into the floor with your wrists and by pulling in your stomach and straightening your arms. If you can keep your balance, straighten your legs so that your feet stretch out in front of you. To do this really well your wrists must be strong and your hands firmly planted on the floor.

HERO
Virasana

A hero is brave and strong, and unflappable in the face of danger. In Hero pose you sit on the floor with a very tall straight spine. Be calm and quiet. You need flexible hips for this: if you are a bit stiff and your bottom doesn't touch the floor put a cushion between your feet to begin with.

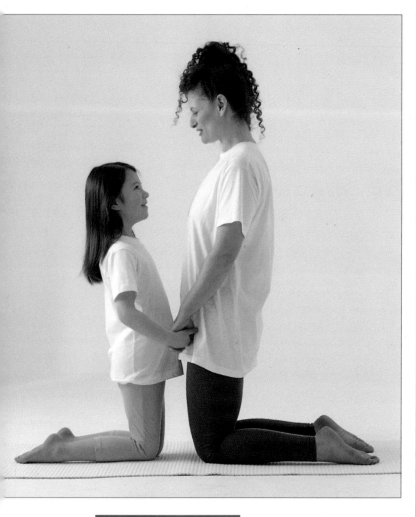

1 Kneel up on a mat or folded blanket, knees together and feet apart.

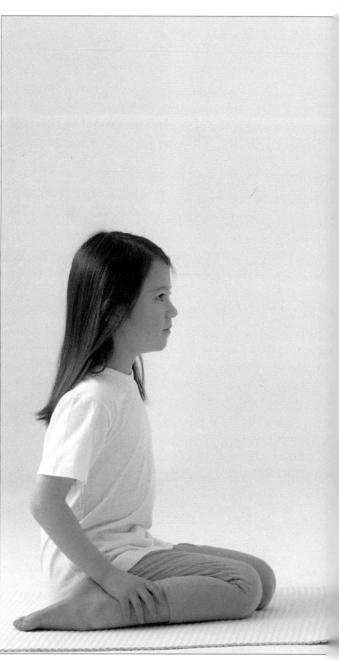

2 Sit between your feet making sure your feet and ankles are straight with toes pointing backwards. Your sitting bones should be resting on the floor.

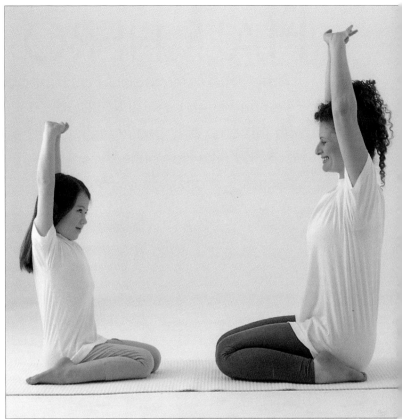

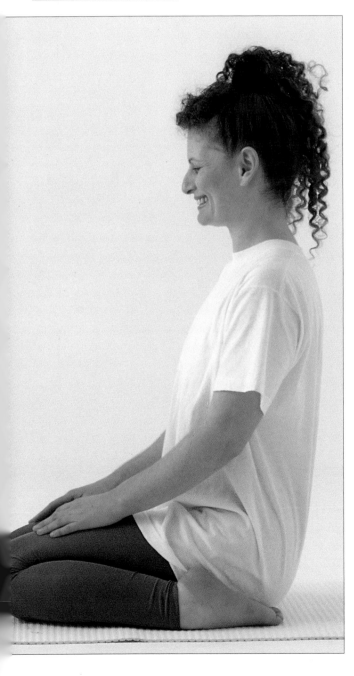

3 Link your fingers together and stretch your arms above your head, turning the palms to the ceiling. Breathing out, keep your hips down so that your spine can lengthen. Don't tighten your shoulders.

HALF HERO
Triang Mukhaikapada Paschimottanasana

If you find Hero pose difficult, start with this one: only one leg is folded back and, like Half Butterfly, it stretches first one side of your body and then the other. One day, when your hips are flexible enough, you will be able to bend forwards very low and flat along the outstretched leg.

1 Sit between your heels, knees together. Put your left leg straight out in front of you, knee facing upwards. Sit tall.

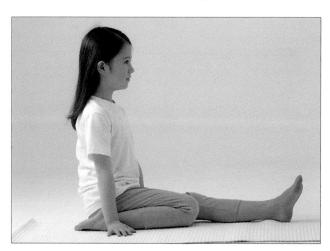

2 Then, as you breathe out, bend forward gently over the straight leg reaching forward with your right arm to touch your toe, and keeping the buttocks of the bent leg on the floor.

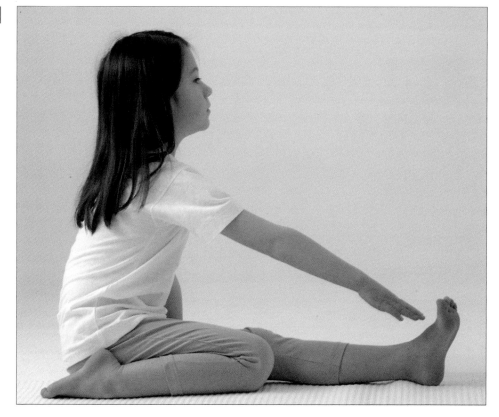

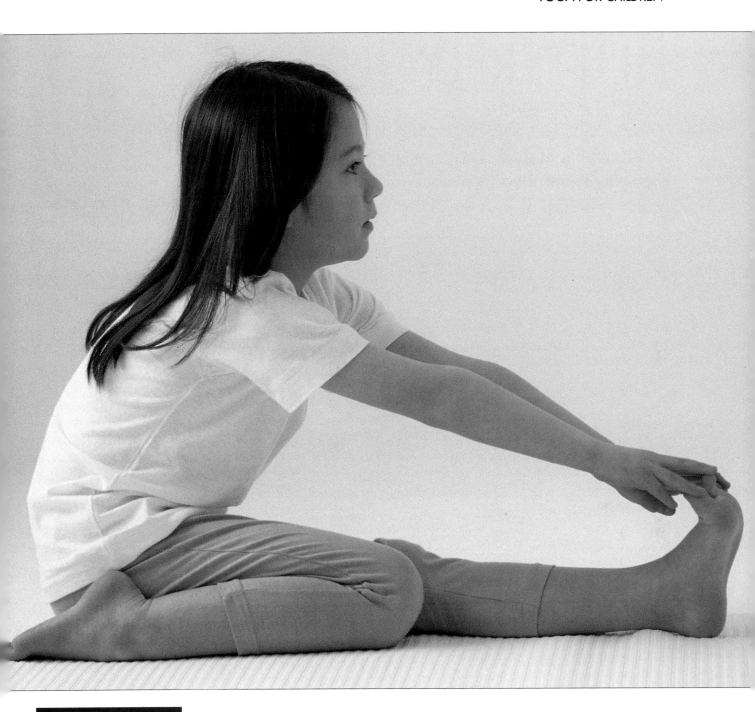

3 Reach forward with both hands. Keep both hips down so that your spine can lengthen forwards. Come up and repeat the pose on the other side.

BUTTERFLY

Baddha Konasana

Imagine a butterfly's wings opening as it emerges from its chrysalis. In a similar way your thighs should turn out and your knees drop down towards the floor.

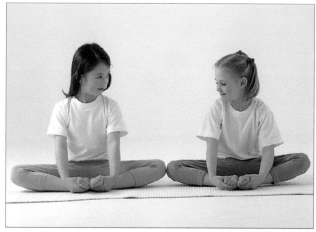

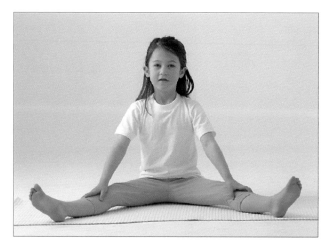

1 Sit on the floor with your legs straight and wide apart. Drop your hips and let your spine grow tall.

2 Bend your knees and pull your feet towards you until the soles touch. Put your hands around your feet so that as your hips go down your spine lengthens. Breathe out and drop your knees down to the floor.

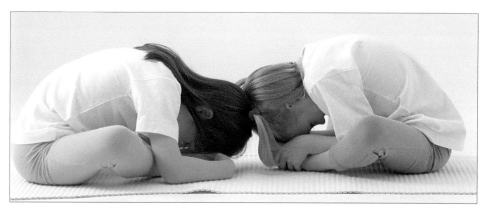

3 Breathe out and bend forward; put your head on the floor in front of you. Keep your hips down so that your back lengthens. Don't pull on your feet, rather let the breathing help your knees drop down.

Turn the soles of the feet up to face the ceiling and you will find that your knees go even further down.

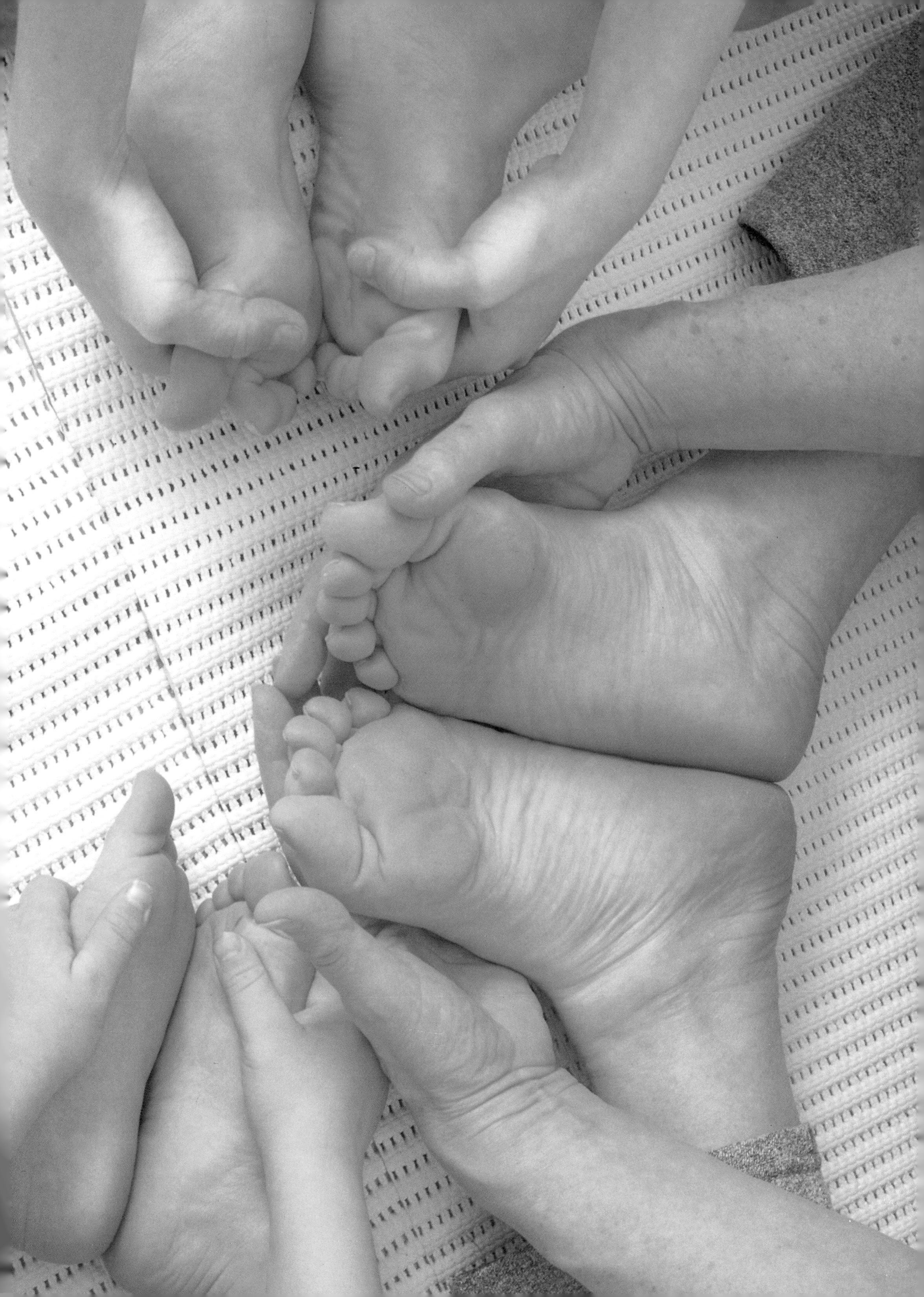

HALF BUTTERFLY

Janu Sirsasana

Sitting in this pose keep one leg straight and bend the other leg as in Butterfly. If Butterfly is difficult for you, practice this one to begin with. It stretches one side of your body first, and then the other side.

1 Sit up very straight with your legs in front of you. Stretch your heels and the backs of your knees. Bend the right leg, bringing your foot to the inside of your left thigh. Let the right leg drop.

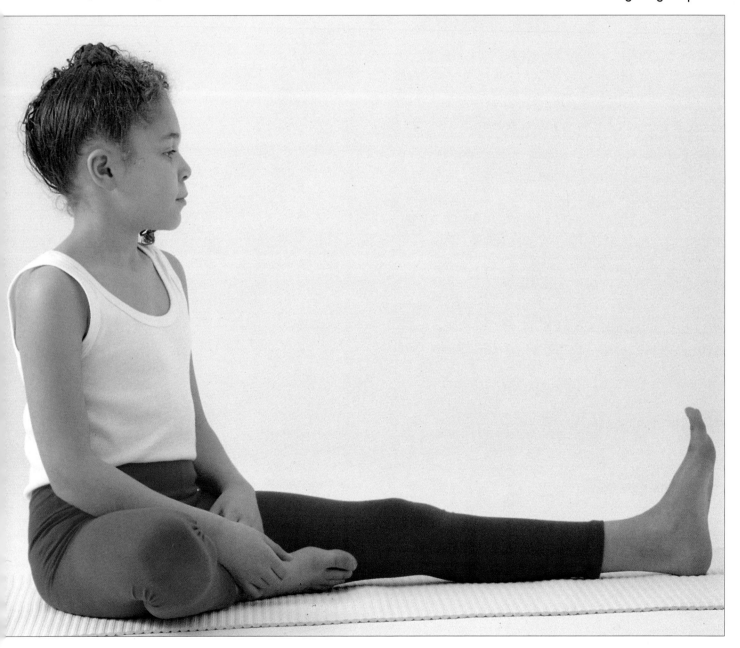

46

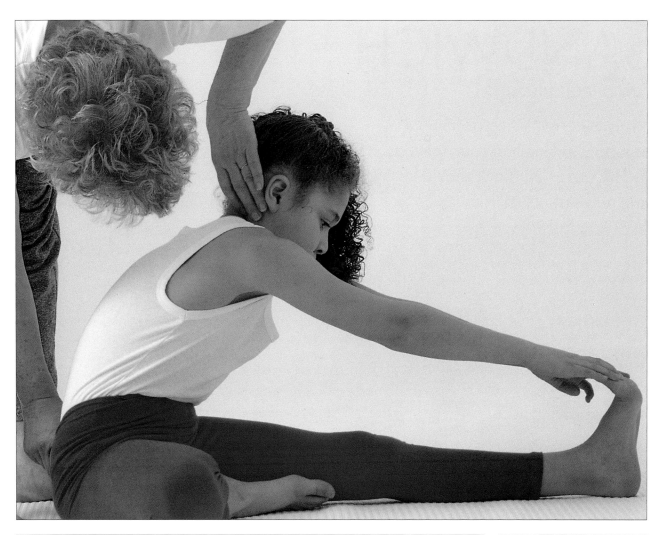

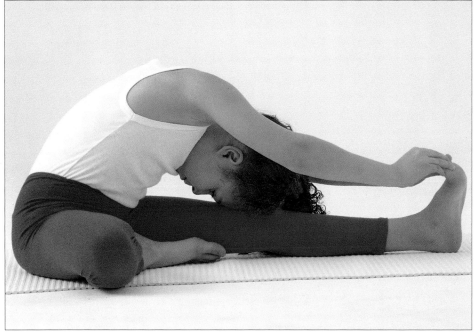

2 Breathe out and keeping both buttocks on the floor, stretch forward and upward from the right hip and catch your left foot with your right hand.

3 Breathe out and stretch further, letting your spine grow longer, but don't pull yourself forward by hanging on to your foot. Repeat with the other knee bent.

SANDWICH
Paschimottanasana

This is the basic sitting position. It's important to lengthen your spine as you go forward - your back should be as long and straight as your legs.

1 Sit on a mat or folded blanket, with your legs straight out in front of you. Sit evenly on both buttock bones with your back long and straight.

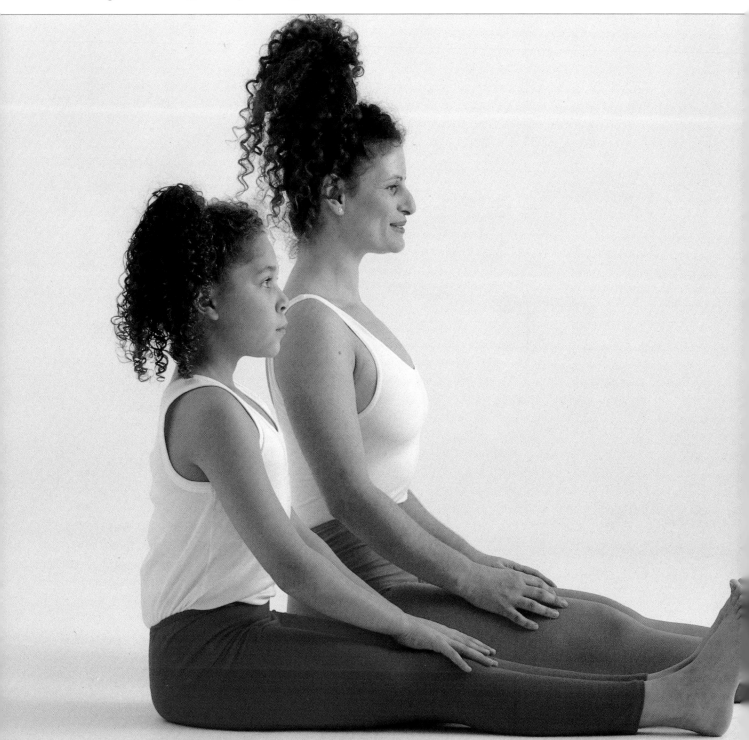

2 Breathe out, stretch forward and catch your feet or big toes. Keep your knees straight. Breathe out and lengthen along your spine. Don't pull on your legs and hunch your back.

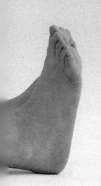

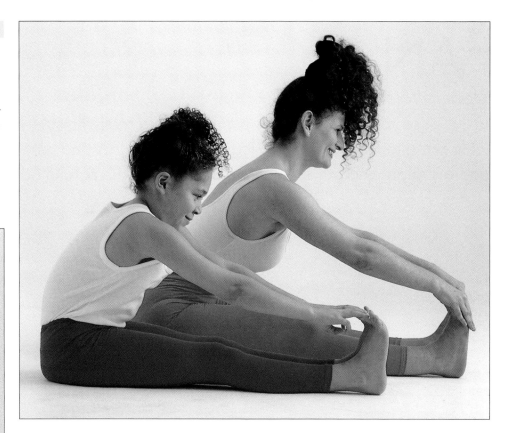

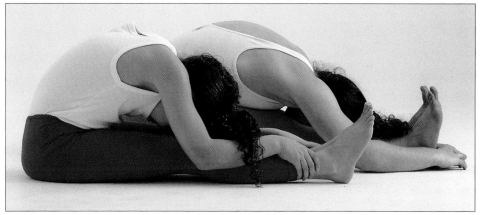

3 Keeping your sitting bones firmly on the floor, breathe out and move your spine forward little by little from its base until eventually you can rest your head on your shins. Don't spoil the Sandwich by letting your knees bend or by pulling on your hands.

FAN

Upavistha Konasana

In this pose you open your legs out wide like a fan. You need long legs and a straight back for it. When you are really flexible you can stretch forwards and put your head on the floor. Be careful not to bend your knees.

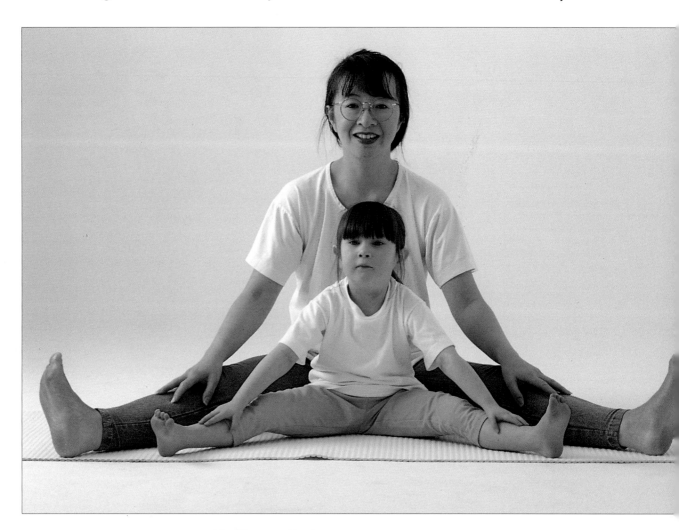

1 Sit with your legs wide apart and the knees straight. Keep your back straight and your shoulders relaxed and down. For some people this first position may be enough of a stretch in itself to begin with.

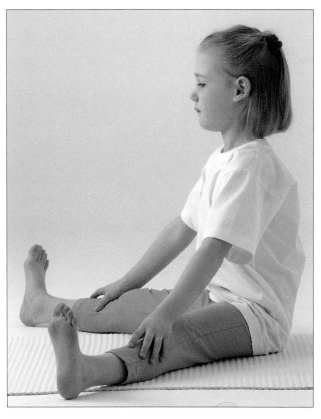

2 Keeping your buttocks on the floor grow tall and see if you can touch your feet. If you can't do this, put your hands on the floor close to your hips, or rest them on your knees and sit up tall - this is far enough for the time being.

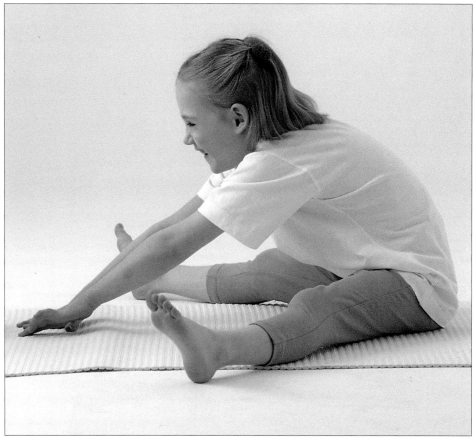

3 Breathe out and grow longer and longer but keep your knees flat on the ground and your back really straight with shoulders relaxed. Now stretch your arms forwards. If you can, go down and rest your head on the floor. Breathe out as you come up again.

BOW & ARROW

Akarna Dhanurasana

This is like an archer drawing a bow. Hold the 'bow' steadily in front of you with one hand; pull back the 'arrow' and 'bowstring' with the other.

1 Sit on the floor with both legs straight out in front of you. Sitting tall, keep your hips down and hold both big toes.

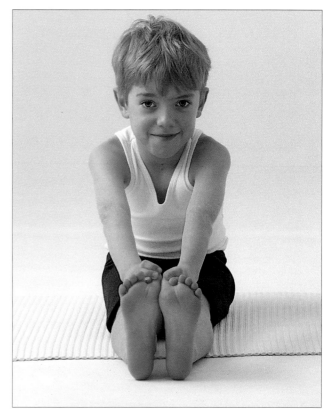

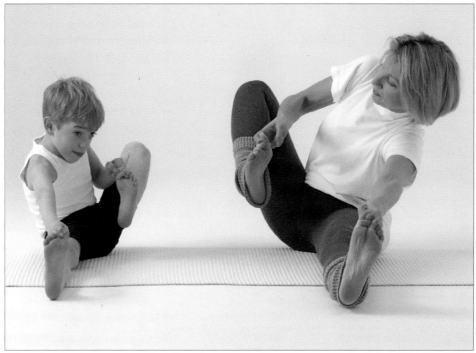

2 Breathe out and, keeping one leg firmly on the floor and continuing to hold your toe, bend the other one and pull your foot towards your ear.

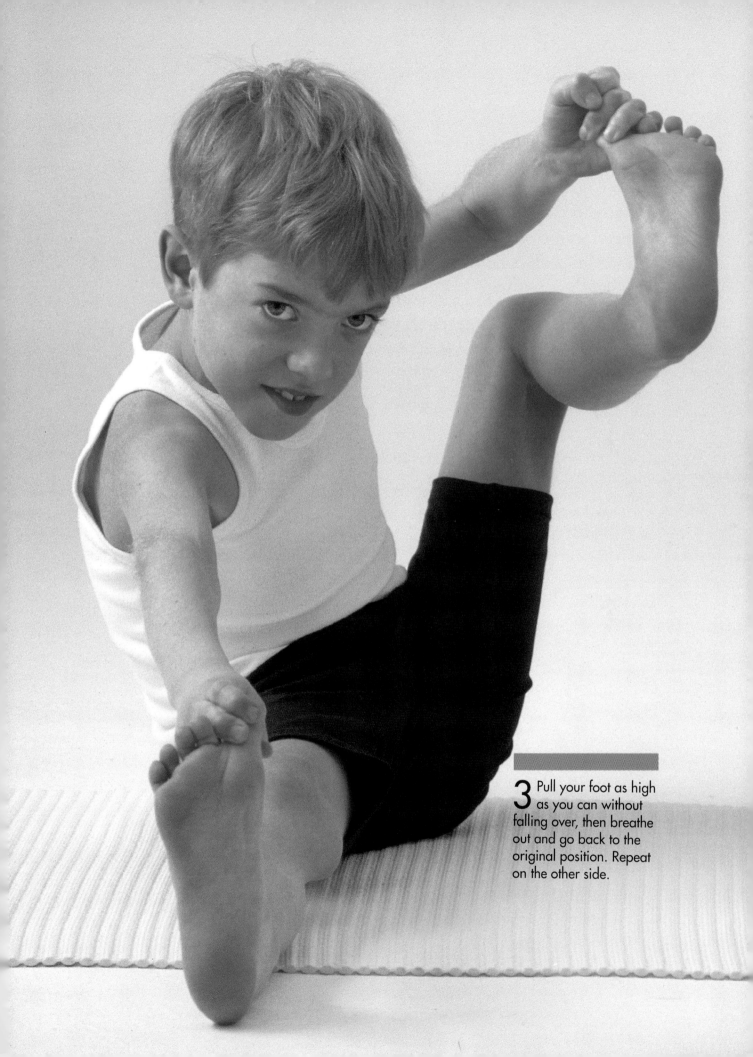

3 Pull your foot as high as you can without falling over, then breathe out and go back to the original position. Repeat on the other side.

Cow

Gomukhasana

This pose is called Cow because the shape of your crossed legs is supposed to resemble a cow's horns. It works the hips and shoulders hard.

1 Sit with your legs simply crossed over each other, then stretch up as straight as you can.

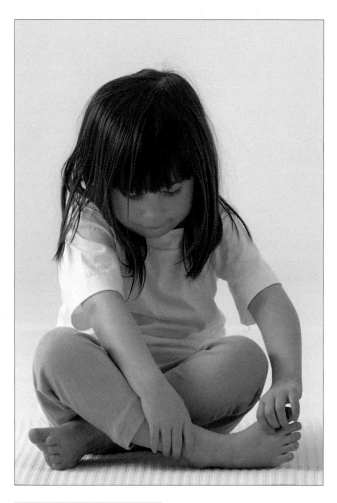

2 Breathe out and cross the legs further so that your knees are one above the other and your feet are on each side of your hips.

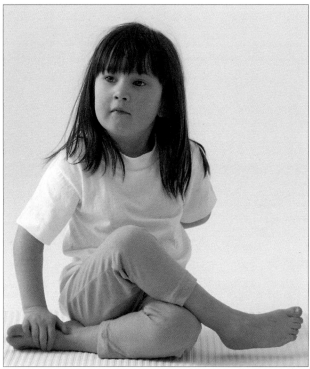

3 Keeping your hips down, sit up tall and take one hand behind your back. Turn it so that the fingers are pointing up between your shoulder blades and the palm is facing out. Breathe out and stretch the other arm up over your head. Bend this top elbow and drop the hand behind your back to clasp the other one.

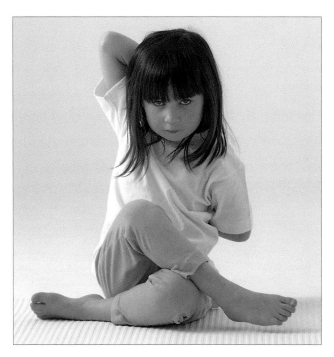

4 Sit up straight, keeping your shoulders relaxed. Release your hands, uncross your legs and do the pose the other way around. It doesn't matter which way your legs are crossed in relation to your arms, as long as you do the pose on both sides.

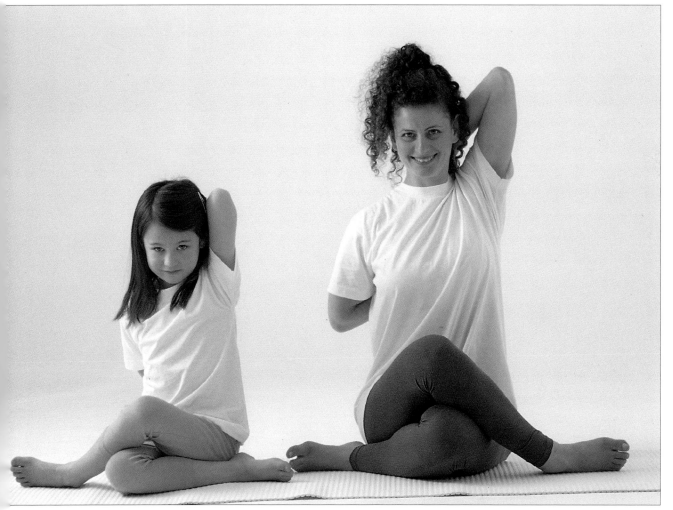

TURTLE
Kurmasana

This pose looks like a tortoise or turtle - the turtle's head and legs are coming out from under the shell, made from your rounded back. Even though your back curves you need to lengthen your spine as you go into the pose.

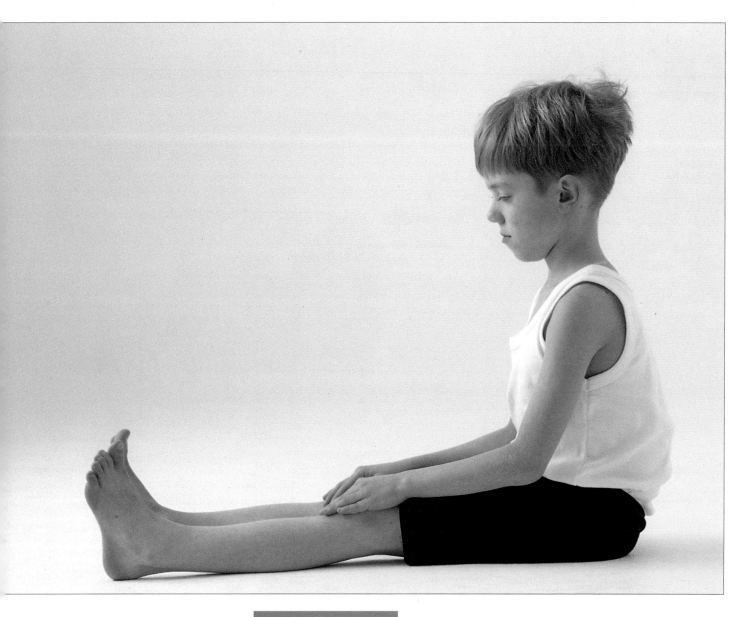

1 Sit on the floor with a straight back, and with your legs straight out in front of you and shoulder width apart. Your toes should be pointing upwards.

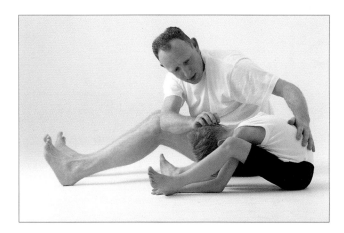

2 Bend your knees and, keeping your hips down, let your spine lengthen forwards so that your arms fall between your legs.

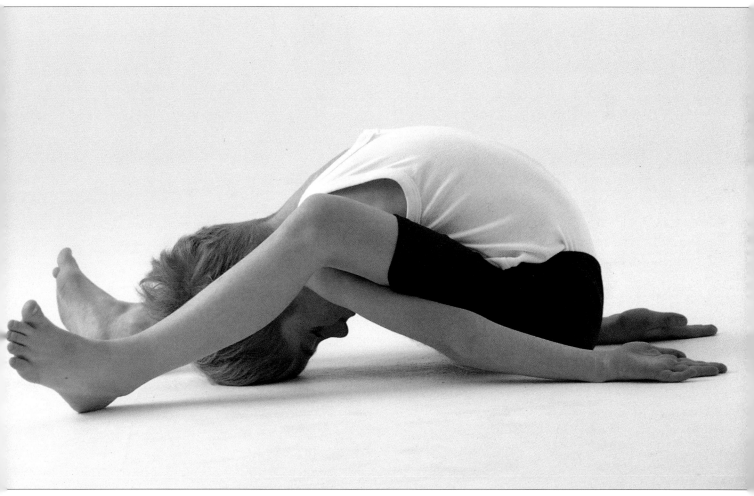

3 Thread each arm through the bended knees one by one. Turn your palms upwards and stretch your hands out behind your hips. Breathe out and straighten your legs as much as you can, stretch your heels and lengthen your back as much as possible. Bend your knees and come up slowly and gently.

SITTING TWIST

Marichyasana

When you are sitting you should be able to twist any way you want. Here you twist around your knee so that you can hold your hands behind your back. If you're flexible and have long arms you can twist around the outside of your leg. There is an easier way for people who are a bit stiffer.

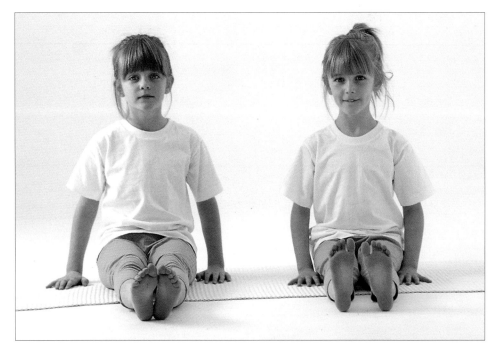

1 Sit up tall on a mat or folded blanket with your legs out in front of you. Sit evenly on both buttock bones, feet parallel and toes pointing upwards.

2 Bend your right knee up close to the chest keeping the other straight and flat to the floor. Hug your knee and sit up tall.

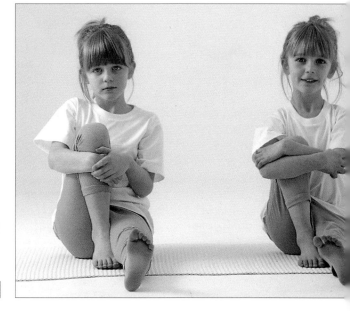

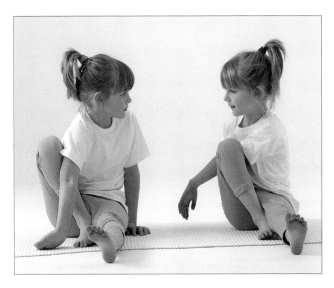

3 Breathe out and turn so that your arm goes around your bent leg. If possible turn so that your left arm goes around the outside of your right leg. If you find this difficult turn the other way, so that your right arm goes around the inside of your right leg.

4 Bend your elbow and turn your arm around your bent leg so that you can clasp your arms behind your back. Sit as tall as you can, then unclasp your hands and do the pose the other way around.

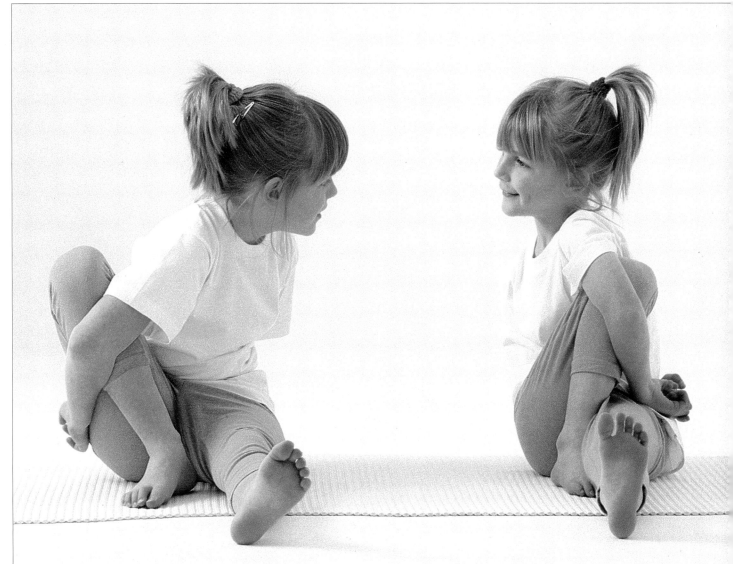

CANDLE

Sarvangasana

This upside-down pose is tall and straight like a candle. Keep your elbows and shoulders firmly on the floor while you grow taller and taller, your feet pointing upwards like the candle flame.

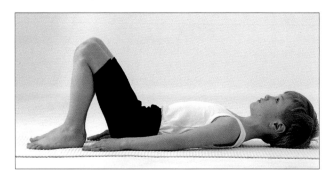

1 Lie flat on a mat, knees bent, arms by your sides, palms down.

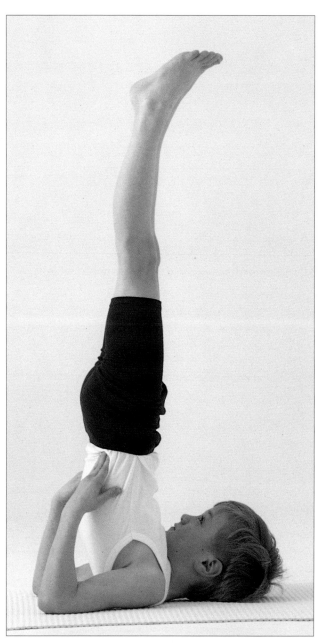

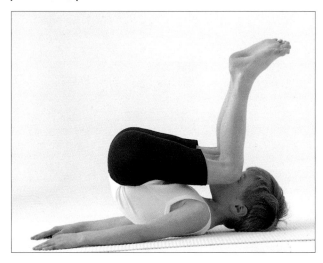

2 Keeping your hands where they are, breathe out and take your legs over your torso. Let your arms drop.

3 Keep your knees bent and place your hands on your back for support. Now raise your hips further, so that you are balanced on the top of your shoulders. Your elbows must stay down on the floor. Uncurl your legs extending them straight up in the air.

60

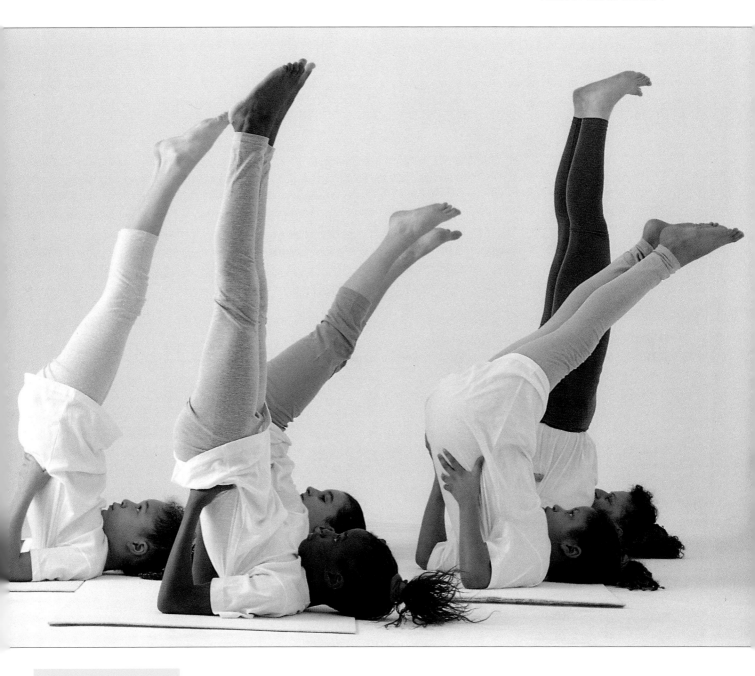

4 Stay in the pose for a few breaths growing taller with each out breath. To come out of the position, bend your knees, put your hands on the floor with the palms flat and roll gently down. When you have learned this you can try some of the variations of Candle, which you can see on the next page.

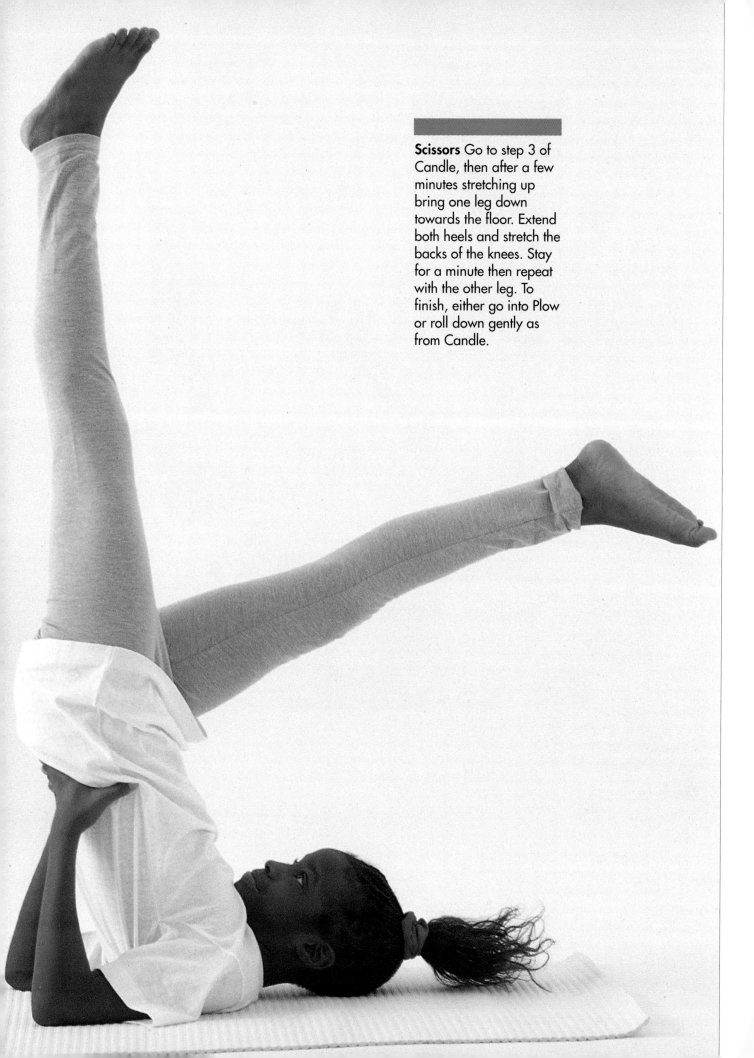

Scissors Go to step 3 of Candle, then after a few minutes stretching up bring one leg down towards the floor. Extend both heels and stretch the backs of the knees. Stay for a minute then repeat with the other leg. To finish, either go into Plow or roll down gently as from Candle.

PLOW
Halasana

Plow follows on from Candle. There are several other variations of Candle, too. Take one leg down into Scissors, or fold your knees up tight on either side of your head like an Accordion.

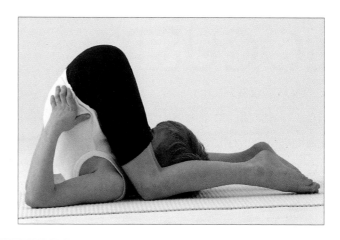

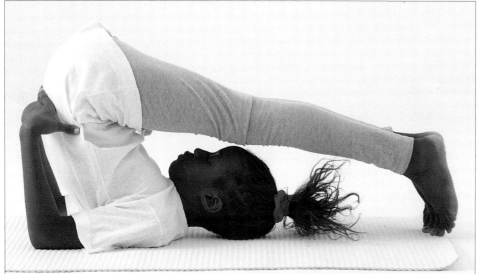

Accordion After step 2 of Candle, breathe out, bend your knees and let them drop towards the floor close to your head.

1 After step 2 of Candle straighten your legs out so that your toes touch the floor. Stretch the backs of your knees and lengthen your body.

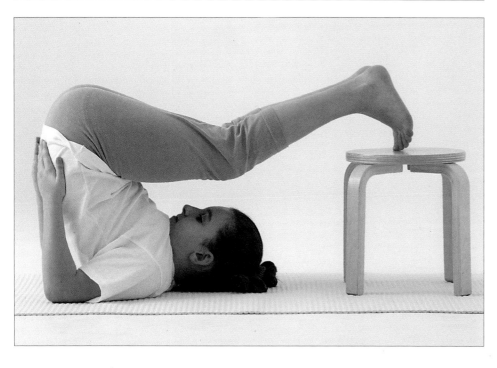

2 If your back collapses when you try to touch your feet to the floor, put your feet on a stool or chair so that your spine can lengthen properly. After you have practiced like this for a few weeks you will be able to touch your feet to the floor quite easily.

LOCUST

Salabhasana

You must learn this simple back bend before you attempt the difficult ones such as Wheel. In all back bends the aim is to lengthen the spine as well as bend it.

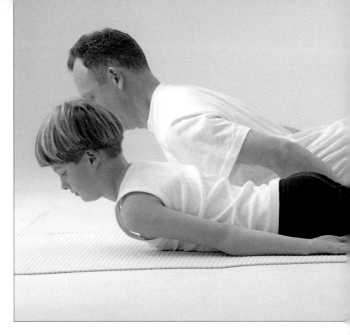

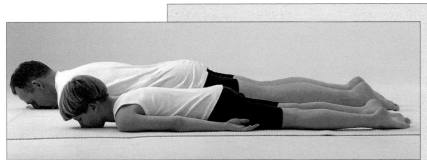

1 Lie flat face down on a mat or folded blanket. Have your arms by your sides with the palms upwards. Breathe out and feel your back go down flatter and flatter into the floor.

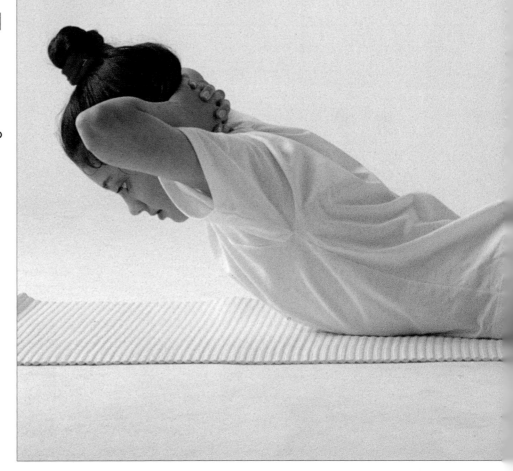

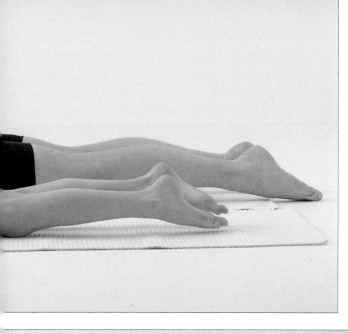

2 Imagine someone is pulling the top of your head forwards with a string so that your spine grows longer and longer, then lift your head and shoulders off the floor.

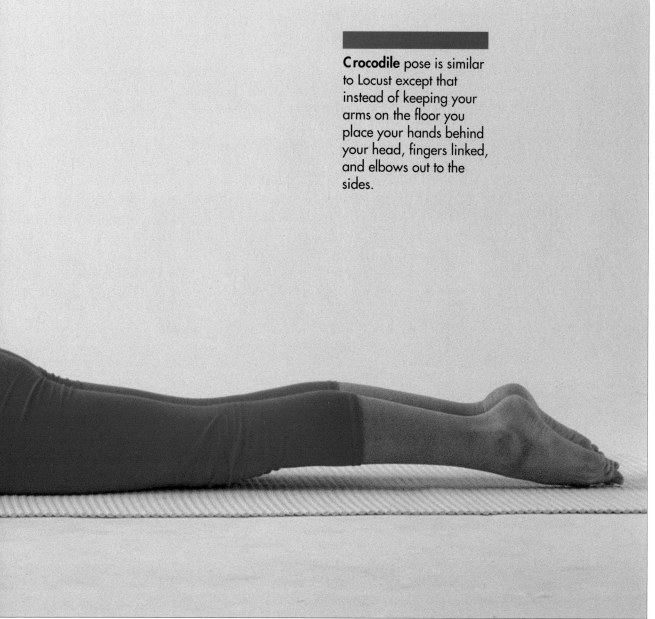

Crocodile pose is similar to Locust except that instead of keeping your arms on the floor you place your hands behind your head, fingers linked, and elbows out to the sides.

SNAKE

Bhujangasana

Here you slide forwards like a snake
and rear your head up as if the snake
was about to strike. Sometimes this pose
is called Cobra, which is a dangerous
snake found in India.

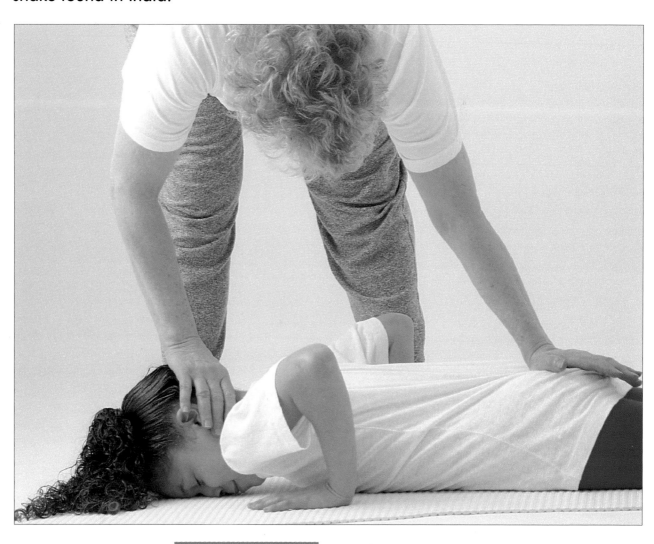

1 Lie flat on a mat or blanket face down with your hands beside your chest. Keep your palms down and your fingers pointing forwards.

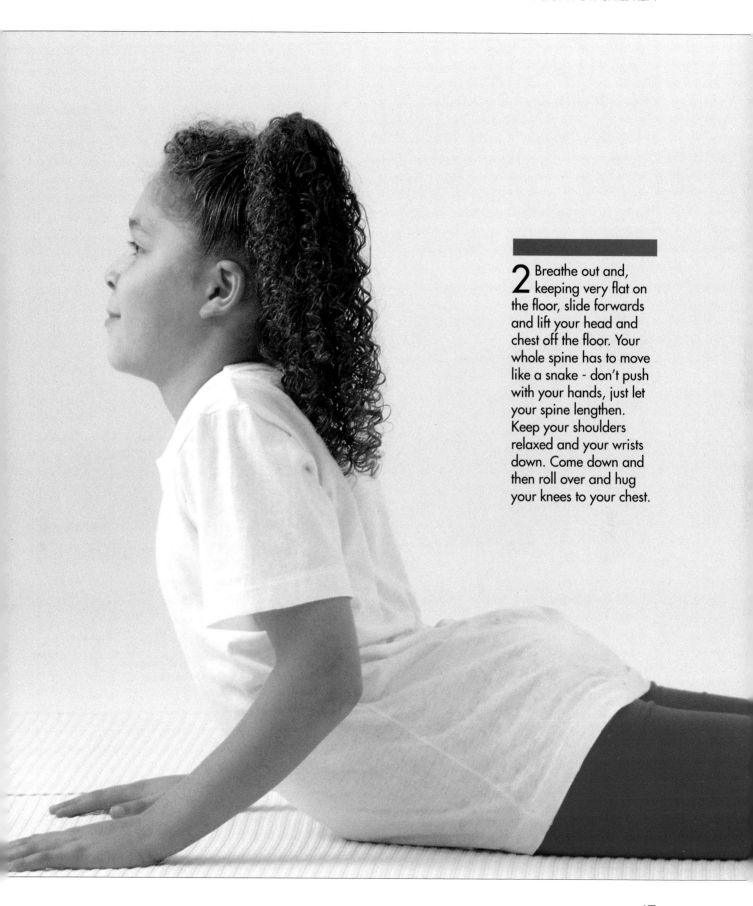

2 Breathe out and, keeping very flat on the floor, slide forwards and lift your head and chest off the floor. Your whole spine has to move like a snake - don't push with your hands, just let your spine lengthen. Keep your shoulders relaxed and your wrists down. Come down and then roll over and hug your knees to your chest.

BRIDGE
Setubandha Sarvangasana

In this back-bending pose you lift your legs up to make a hump-backed bridge. Both the elbows and the heels have to be firmly anchored to the floor.

1 Lie on your back with your arms by your sides and your knees bent. Place your feet on the floor close to your hips, toes pointing forwards.

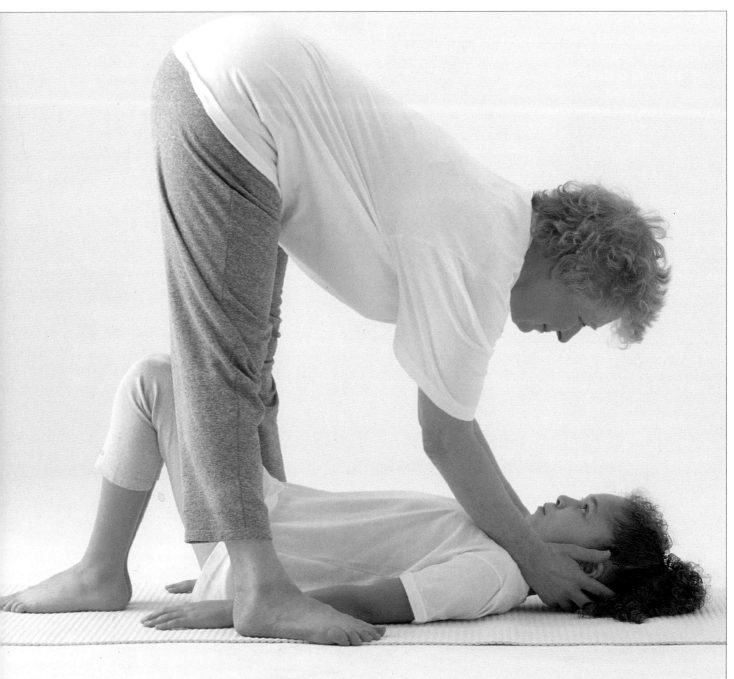

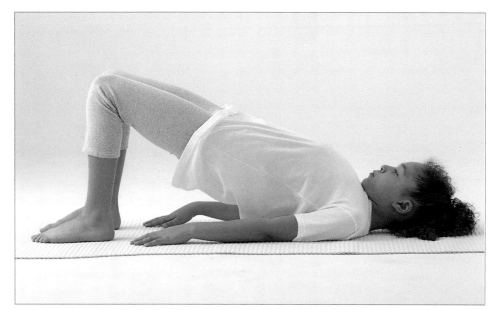

2 Breathe out, drop the back of your waist, then lift your hips up as far as they will go. Keep your heels down on the floor.

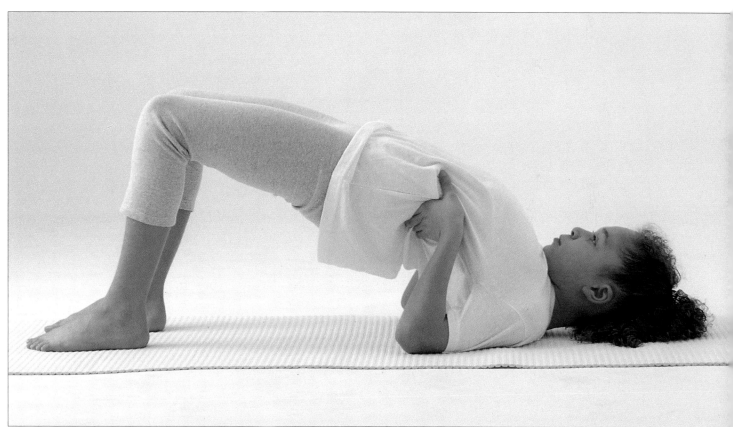

3 Support your back with your hands as in Candle pose. Come down gently and hug your knees to your chest.

WHEEL

Urdhva Dhanurasana

The Wheel is one of the most important and envigorating poses. The back should bend into a round curve so that the whole spine lengthens and does not just hinge at the waist.

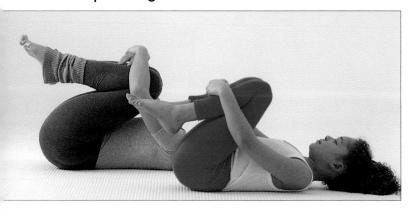

1 Lie on your back on the floor on a non-slip mat. Hug your knees towards you, keeping your chin tucked in. This makes sure that your back is long at the back of your waist before you start the pose.

2 Drop your feet to the floor close to your hips. Your feet must be parallel and your heels down. Lift your arms over your head and place palms by the shoulders with fingers pointing towards the feet.

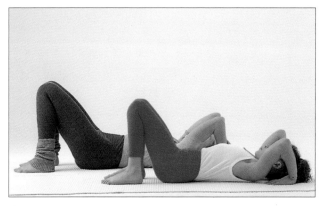

To stop your feet splaying out in this pose you can do it with a belt round your thighs above your knees.

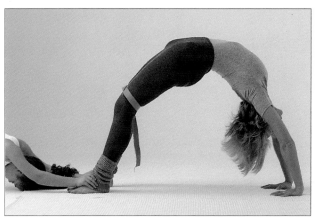

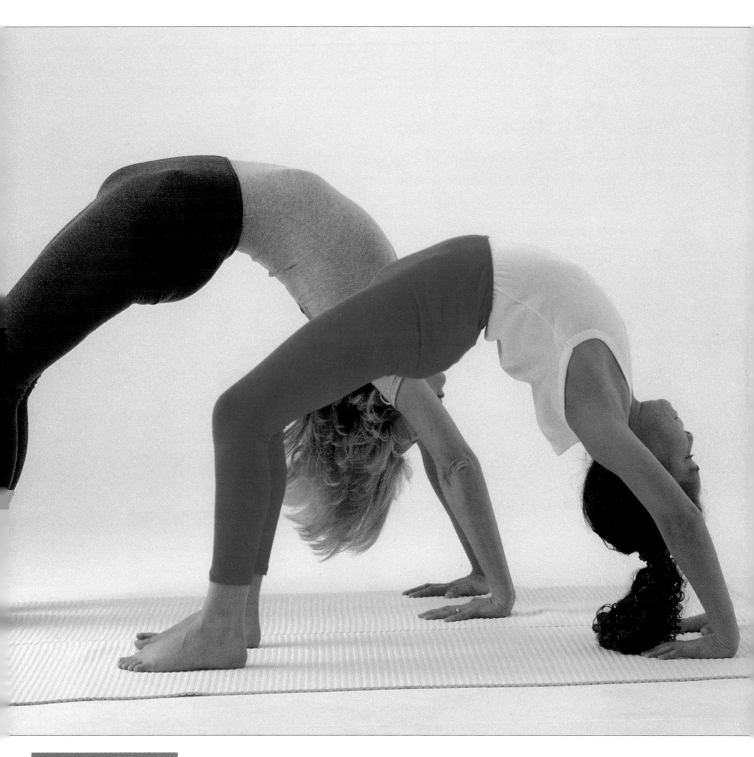

3 Breathe deeply and relax. Breathe out and, keeping the back of the waist long, lift up into the pose with the impetus of the out-breath. Keep your heels down as you go up, and your feet parallel. As you stay in the pose, let your back lengthen as you breathe out. Your whole spine should feel free, with no pressure in the back of your waist. Come down and hug your knees as in step 1.

SUNDANCE

Surya Namaskar

This is a cycle of familiar movements which should be practiced in sequence. It is a greeting and salutation to the sun - a coordination of body, breath and attention. Traditionally, it is repeated 12 times, once for each month of the year.

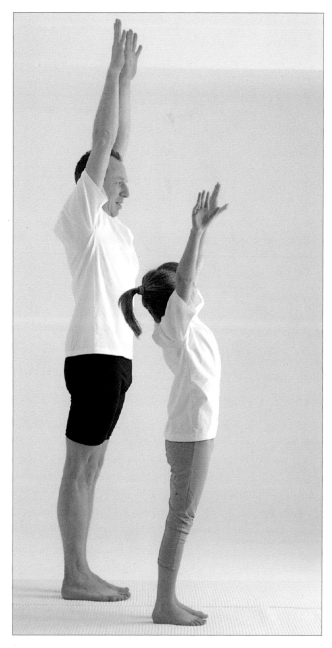

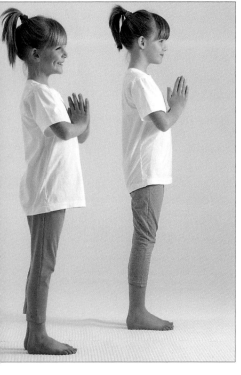

1 Stand straight and tall with your elbows bent and the palms of your hands together.

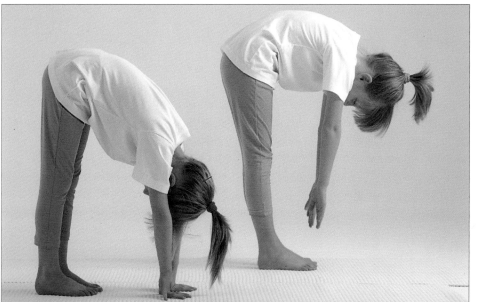

2 Breathe in and raise your arms above your head.

3 Breathe out. Bend over from your hips as in Rag Doll (page 22). Keep your heels down.

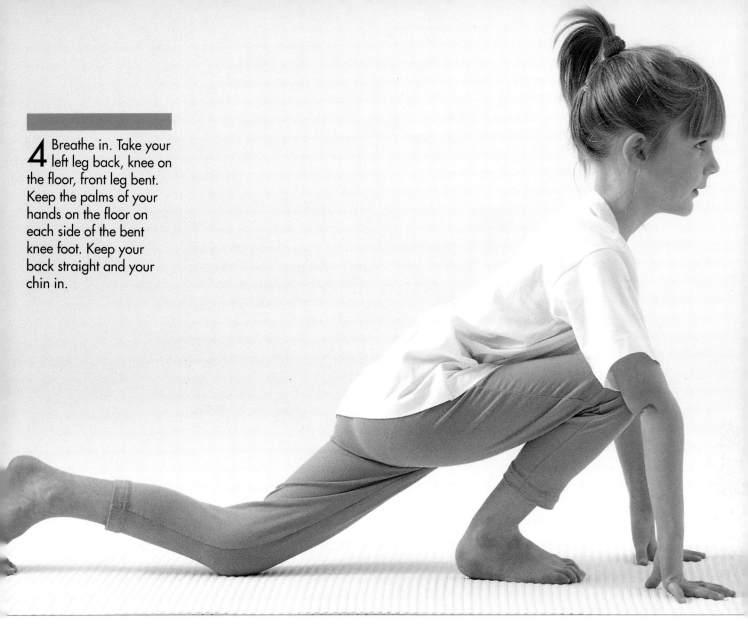

4 Breathe in. Take your left leg back, knee on the floor, front leg bent. Keep the palms of your hands on the floor on each side of the bent knee foot. Keep your back straight and your chin in.

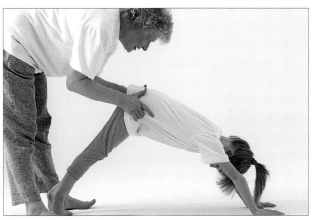

5 Breathe out. Keep your hands where they are and swing the front leg back to join the other. Lift up your hips and move into Dog pose (page 32) with your legs straight and back long. Keep your heels down.

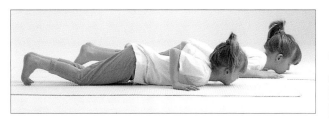

6 Breathe in. Breathe out and bend your elbows. Keeping your bottom up slide forward between your hands.

SUNDANCE

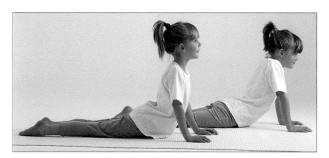

7 Breathe in. Raise your head, straighten your arms and drop your hips and legs. This is Snake pose (page 66).

8 Breathe out and go back into Dog pose (step 5) by leaving your hands where they are and lifting your hips up and back. Keep your heels down.

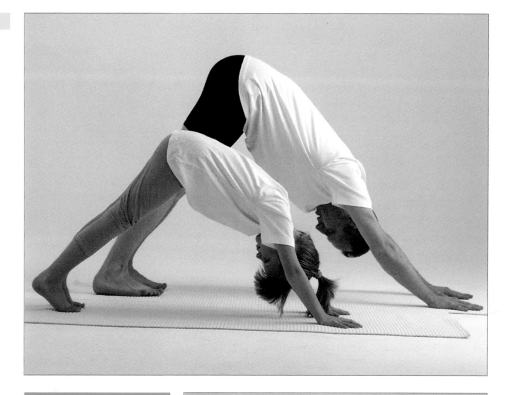

9 Breathe in. Take the left leg forward. The front knee is bent and the back leg knee touches the floor.

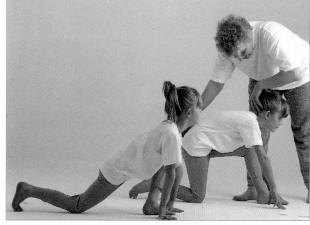

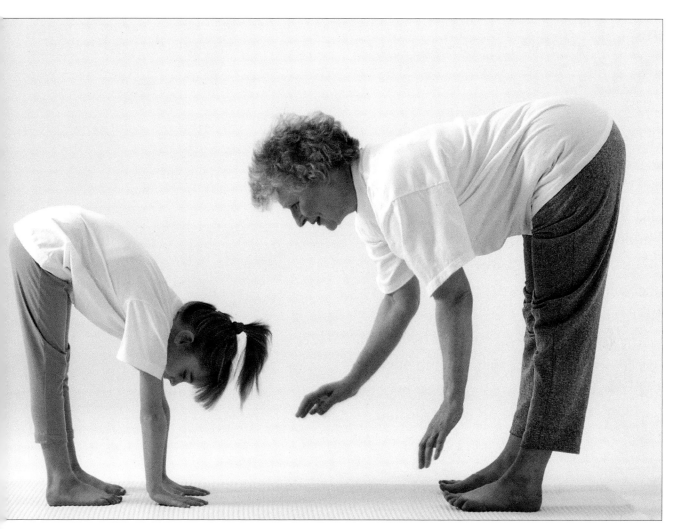

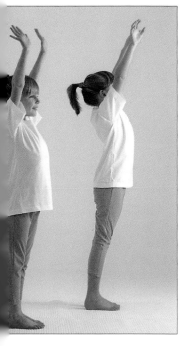

10 Breathe out. Bring your right leg forward so that the feet are parallel (*above*), and fold forward from the hips as in step 3.

11 Breathe in. Lift up your trunk (*left*), keeping your weight on your heels, and raise your arms above your head in one smooth movement.

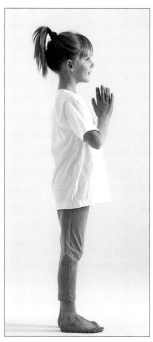

12 Breathe out. Bend your elbows, place the palms of your hands together in prayer position (*left*) and stand up straight and tall as in the starting pose.

REST

Stillness and quiet are just as important as action and movement. But in a noisy and frenetic world it can be difficult to find the time and space to wind down. Children are bombarded with stimuli of all kinds and frequently end up becoming just as tense and stressed as their parents.

Yoga exercises can help them rediscover the joy of stillness and silence and teach them how to breathe evenly, and how to be quiet and concentrated.

Lying flat on your back with your arms across your chest and knees bent up helps you relax and melt into the floor. Keep your head straight.

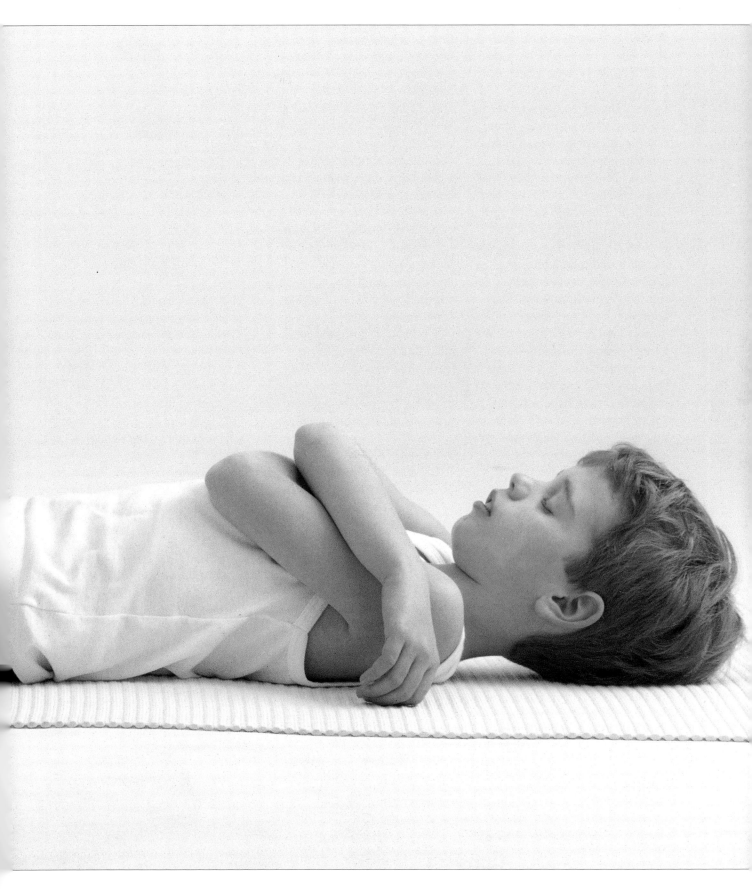

The body needs rest as much as it needs action. Restful poses and breathing are an essential part of every yoga practice session. They should always follow the more strenuous poses. When doing yoga with groups of children the most popular part of the session has always been the quiet time at the end. Children respond well to this chance to be still and silent even if it is only for a few minutes. Their minds are open and receptive and a time of quiet allows them to develop their creativity and individuality. Tiny fidgety children and teenagers with examination nerves can all benefit.

Interestingly, children whose concentration span is short seem to have a better capacity for staying still and quiet than many adults. Adults have often lost the ability to stay quiet and find themselves self-conscious and insecure when asked to stay silent in a group.

STILLNESS AND SILENCE
Restful poses and games in yoga are in complete contrast to the general pattern of a child's life. The pace today is fast and increasingly noisy. From the rush and hurly burly of breakfast, the journey to work or school, the demands of a busy day, to the return home, television, homework and socializing, there is little or no time for silence. It has become a precious commodity that is fast disappearing.

More disturbing still is the fact that modern technology has helped to speed up the way we live our

Curling up in Mouse (page 82) is the best way to quieten down a number of children towards the end of a group yoga practice session.

lives. We now all do several things at once. It seems quite normal to eat breakfast, read the newspaper and listen to music at the same time. Children watch television while eating, read while travelling and even choose to plug into their Walkmans as they exercise. High technology has resulted in children being bombarded with distractions.

More distractions and more noise result in more stress and tension. In less crowded times and in more rural environments the chance for moments of peace came easily.

Nowadays, it is good for children to learn to listen to themselves as well as to other people. We need to make a space for quiet and also for stillness. We have to fight for tranquillity.

WINDING DOWN
To become still and silent you first have to wind down. Generally, when you practise yoga you wind down towards the end of the session and end up lying flat on the floor in the Dead Man's Pose (page 96). With children the sessions are not so long, so in this chapter there are several ideas for

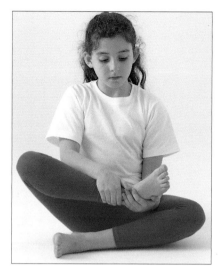

Lotus pose (page 88) is a classic yoga position. By sitting straight and centred, you become still and quiet and able to focus inward.

quietening down just before relaxation that can either be used at the end of the class or for a few minutes quiet before children go to bed.

Flopping, stretching and breathing exercises are ideal ways of winding down.

BREATHING
Breathing is versatile. It can be used to wake you up, and to quieten you down, and just in general to help you relax and get

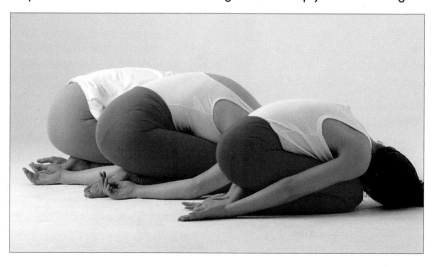

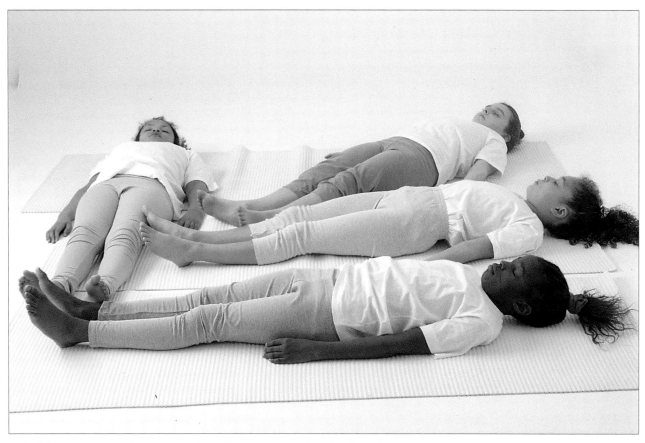

rid of the stresses and tensions of modern life.

Learning about breathing is useful at any age. Even very young children can be taught to breathe evenly. They will discover how the way they breathe affects the way they sit, stand and stretch.

The rhythm of your breathing affects the functioning of all the systems of the body. The main muscle used in breathing is the diaphragm, which lies across your trunk at the bottom of the ribs. When you get out of breath your shoulders and neck muscles help to lift up your ribs when you breathe in, so that your lungs can take in more air. Your lungs are like two sponges or balloons: they expand when you fill them full of air and contract as they empty..

Tension and anxiety, as well as bad posture can affect the way you

breathe. People who breathe too much in the upper chest can often feel anxious and easily exhausted. Yoga teaches you to breathe deeply and steadily. It counteracts the negative effects of strain and stress.

Using the breath in different ways - buzzing, yawning, blowing and sighing - helps to release tension. Breathing in restful poses and simple stretching can teach children invaluable lessons in how to relax.

FOCUSSING INWARDS
It is important for children to find some time in which to enjoy complete calm in the absence of noise and distraction.

This period of quiet is also necessary to teach them how to refocus their energies and recharge their batteries. They don't

Lying completely flat on the floor in Dead Man's Pose (page 96) at the end of a yoga class provides the time and space to be silent. This is even more important when you have been working in a large group.

need complicated meditation techniques. In fact, some meditation techniques can be harmful. Just a few minutes of peace and quiet, of withdrawing their attention from outside stimuli and concentrating on what is going on inside, is all that is needed.

Yoga rest positions will encourage children to be still and quiet and to focus their attention inwards. Learning to draw on an inner centre of calm and stability will provide them with an invaluable source of strength throughout their lives.

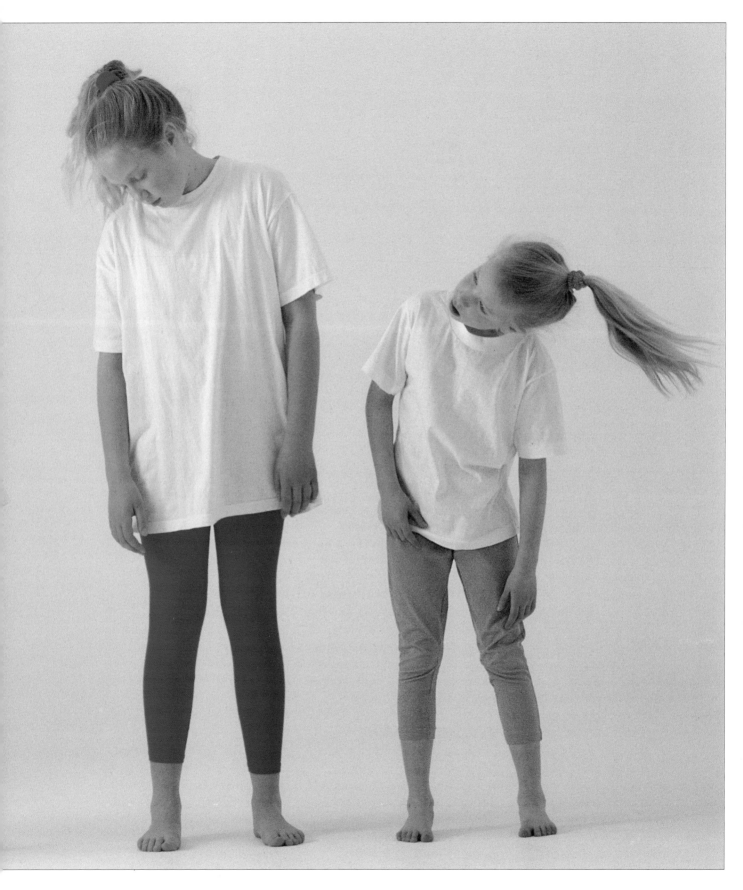

FLOPPING

Flopping is a way of letting go at the end of a session before it's time to relax and become quiet. It can also be used to warm up before you start. There are several ways of doing this either standing or sitting.

Stand straight, raise your arms (*right*) and let them drop heavily so that they swing up again. Let your head and shoulders flop in all directions keeping your feet glued to the floor (*left*). To flop from sitting (*below*), keep your hips down and heavy so that your spine can move easily.

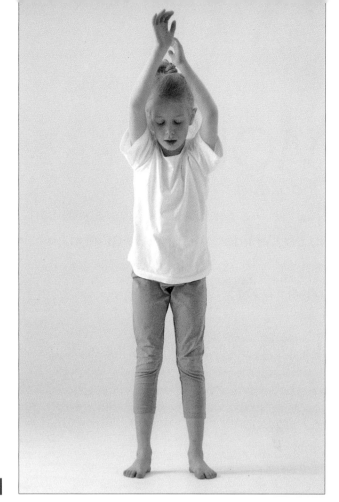

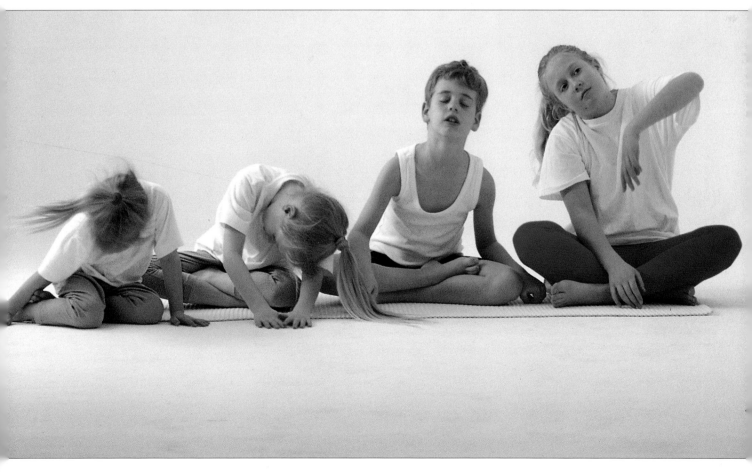

MOUSE

Pindasana

This is a very small pose where you curl up on the floor and stay as quiet as a mouse in its hole. Some people call it 'child's pose'.

1 Kneel on a mat with your knees and feet together. Your toes should point backwards and your heels should touch each other.

2 Sit down on your heels. Your two buttock bones should touch the floor evenly. Sit tall, shoulders relaxed.

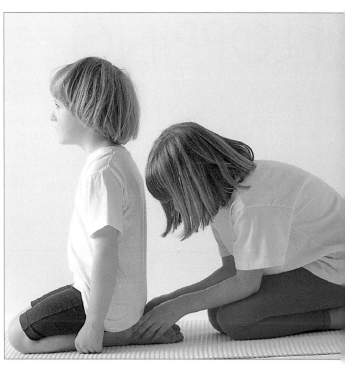

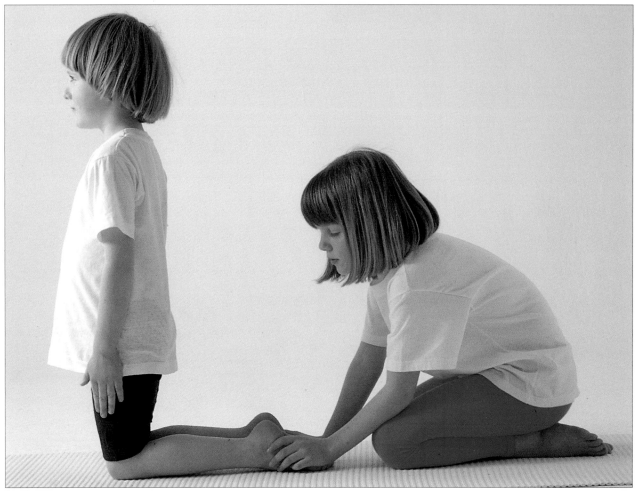

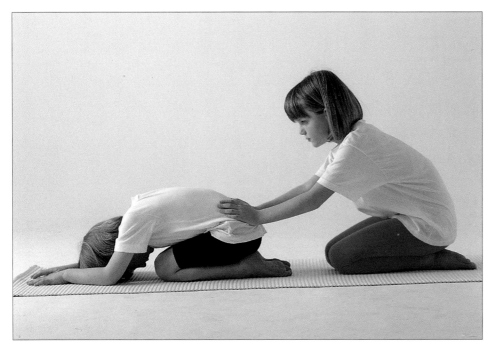

3 Breathe out and slowly lower your torso forward until your head touches the floor. Keep your bottom on your heels. Stretch your arms in front of you.

4 Each time you breathe out let your chest go closer to your knees. Keep shoulders relaxed and take your arms back so your hands are close to your feet.

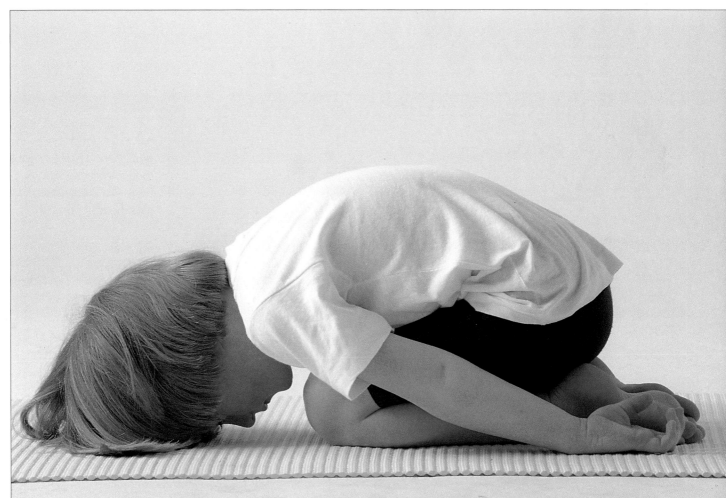

SNOOZE

Yoga Nidrasana

If you can really curl up in this position with your feet behind your head, it is a resting pose. Your feet are a pillow and your legs keep you warm like a blanket.

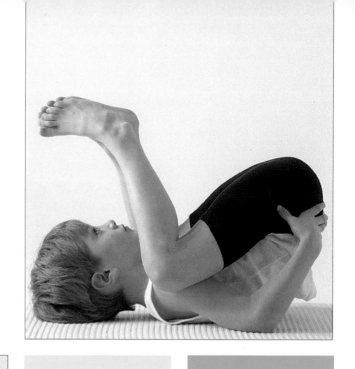

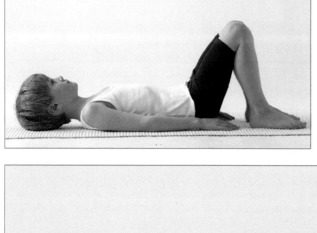

1 Lie on your back with your knees bent up. Keep your head straight and your shoulders relaxed.

2 Breathe out and lift up your hips and bring your feet towards your head.

3 Catch your feet with your hands and gently bring them down to the floor beyond your head. Tuck them behind your head if you can.

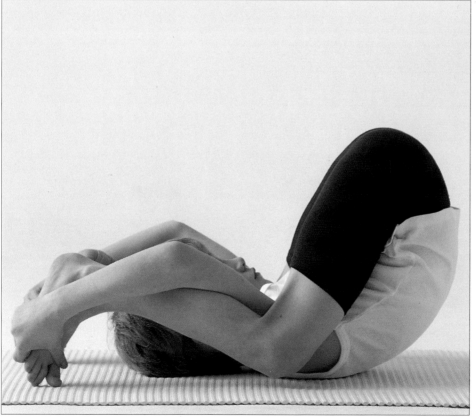

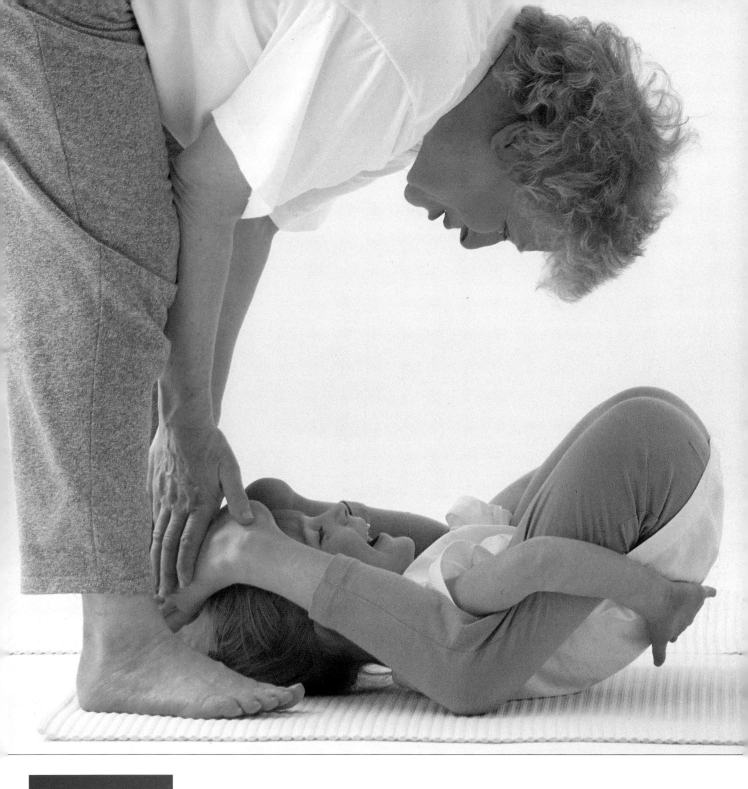

4 Let go your feet. Breathe out and turn your arms and wrap them around your thighs and clasp your hands behind your back.

DIAMOND

Vajrasana

A diamond is a hard stone and this sitting pose has a strong firm base. It helps you to be completely quiet, still and concentrated so that your mind can be clear and sharp as a diamond. You can also practice breathing in this pose.

1 On a folded blanket or mat kneel with your feet together. Sit down on your heels. The heels should be touching each other, toes pointed back, and your bottom should rest on them evenly. Sit up tall and straight.

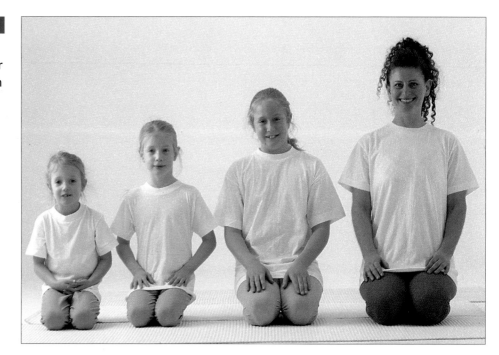

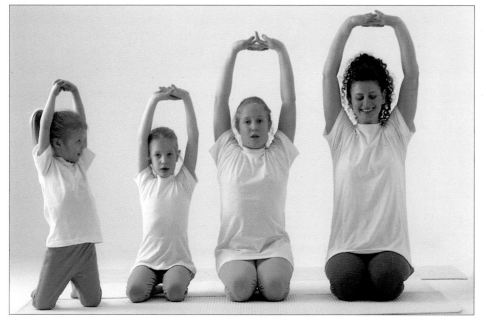

2 You can use this basic sitting position to work your shoulders by stretching your arms up above your head as in Hero pose (page 40).

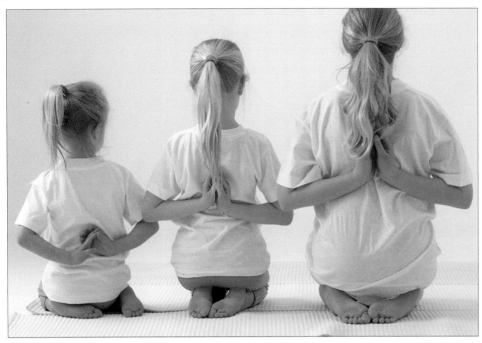

3 You can also stretch your shoulders another way. Put your palms together behind your back with the fingers pointing upwards.

4 To stretch the soles of your feet, turn your toes underneath as you sit on your heels.

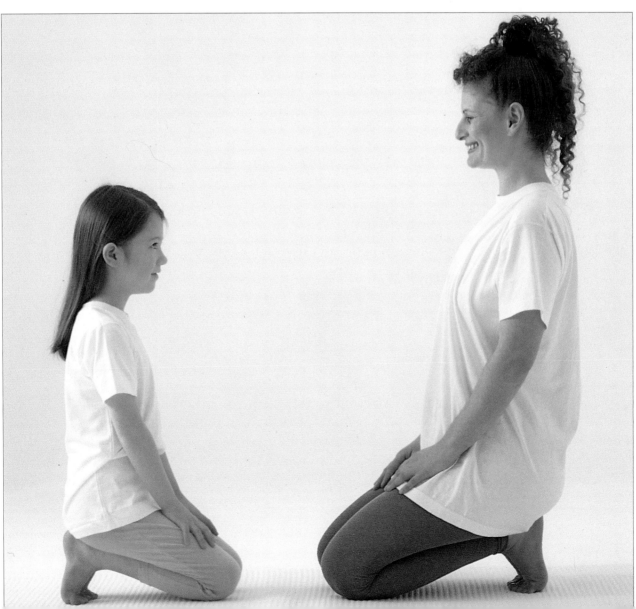

LOTUS
Padmasana

The lotus flower has its roots in the mud.
Despite this the stem rises through the
water and produces a beautiful flower in
the sunlight. In Lotus pose you should sit
straight and centred like the flower.

1 Sit up straight on a
mat or folded blanket
with your legs crossed.
Breathe calmly and
evenly.

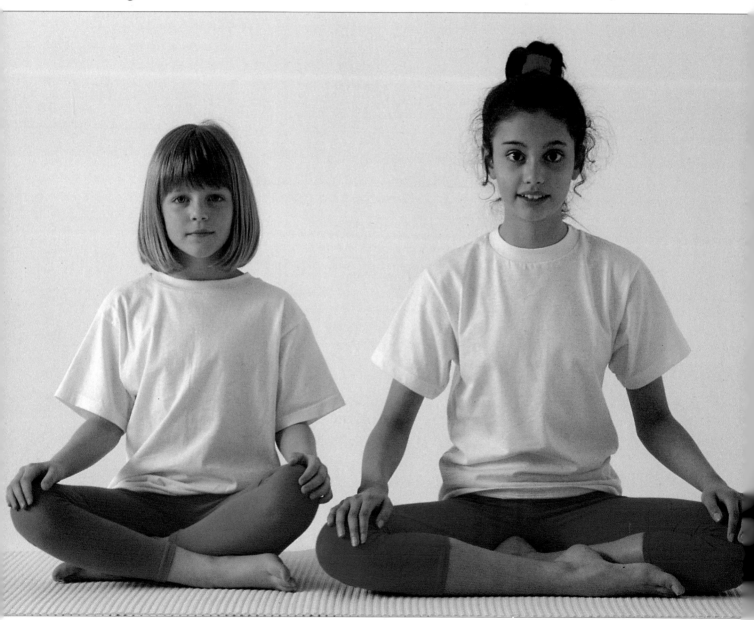

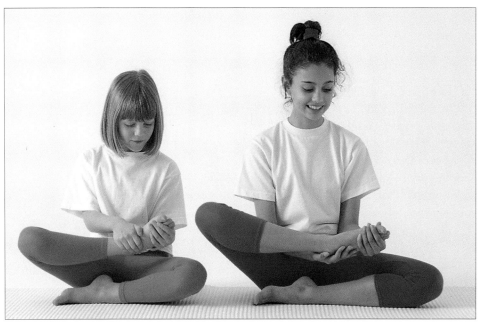

2 Keeping both hips down, breathe out, bend your right knee and lift up your right foot.

3 Place your right foot high up on your left thigh. Let both knees drop to the floor. Keeping your hips down, let your spine grow tall. This is Half Lotus pose. Full Lotus is shown on the next page.

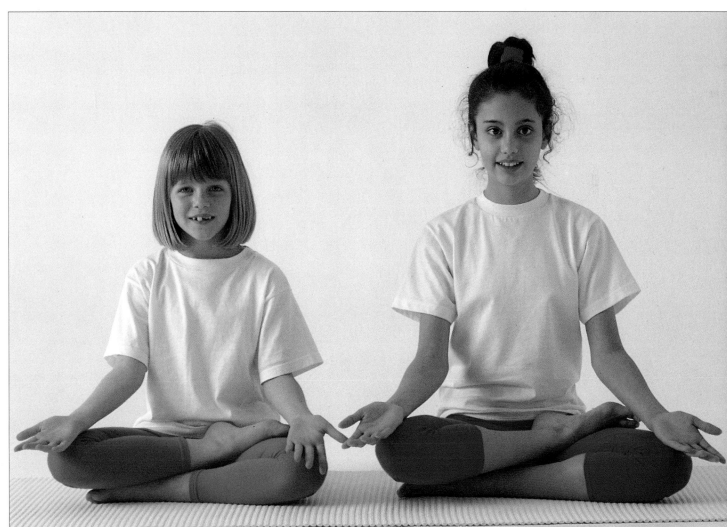

LOTUS

4 To go into Full Lotus from Half Lotus (*previous page*), sit up tall and relax your hips, thighs and shoulders. Keeping your right knee down on the floor, lift up your left foot.

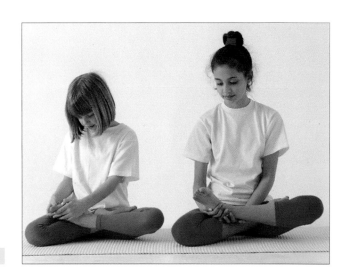

5 Place your left foot as high up on your right thigh as you can. Let both knees drop towards the floor. Your feet will anchor your hips down so that both buttock bones are firmly on the floor and you can sit up tall with your shoulders relaxed. Keep your head straight with the back of your neck long. Repeat with your legs crossed the opposite way.

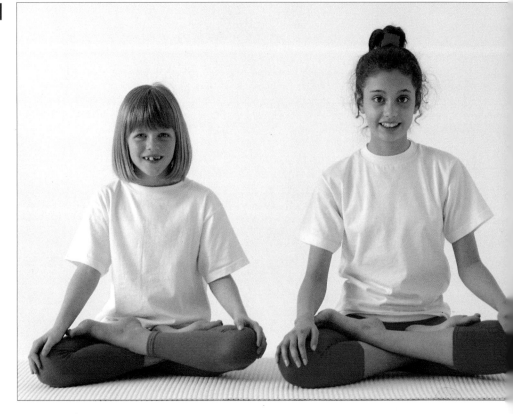

Lotus Forward Bend
From Full Lotus keep your hips down, breathe out and stretch forwards, lengthening your back as you go down.

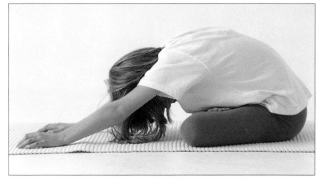

Lotus Twist Sit in Full Lotus pose with your left foot on top. Keep your hips down as you breathe out and turn to the left. Keep your shoulders relaxed and your back tall. Take your left hand behind your back to hold your left foot. Rest your right hand on your left knee. Repeat the pose turning to the other side.

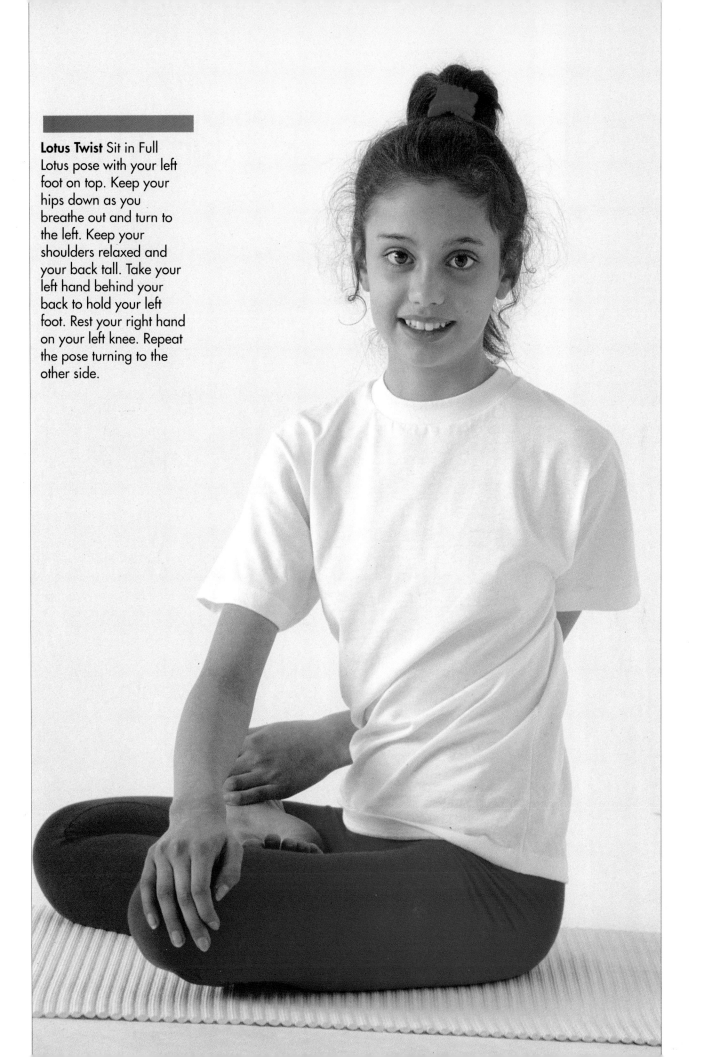

FINDING YOUR BREATH

Discover what happens to your body when you're breathing: what happens to your ribs, your stomach and your shoulders. See how it makes a difference if you're breathing quickly or slowly.

Right Sit up straight and place your hands very gently on your partner's back. Feel the ribcage getting larger and smaller as the breath goes in and out.

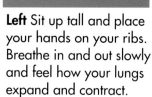

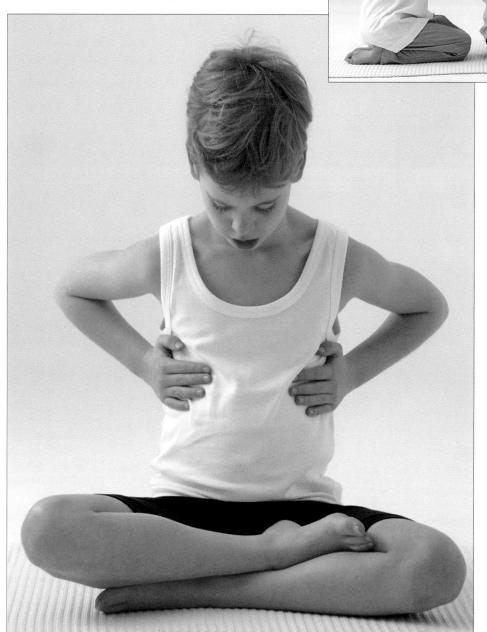

Left Sit up tall and place your hands on your ribs. Breathe in and out slowly and feel how your lungs expand and contract.

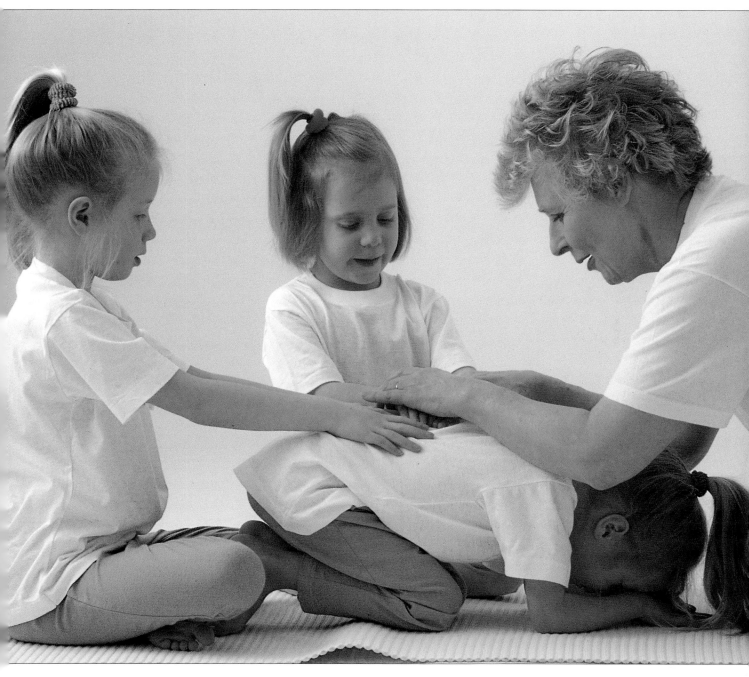

Above Bend forwards in Mouse (page 82) and let your back expand as you breathe in, and get smaller as you breathe out. With their hands on your back, others will be able to feel this, too. Take turns to be Mouse.

Right Put your hand on your stomach and feel it moving as you breathe. As you breathe out it goes in. As you breathe in it goes out.

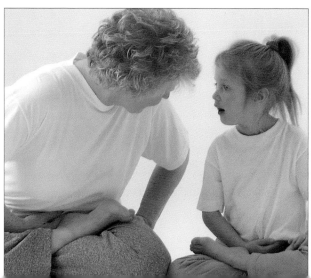

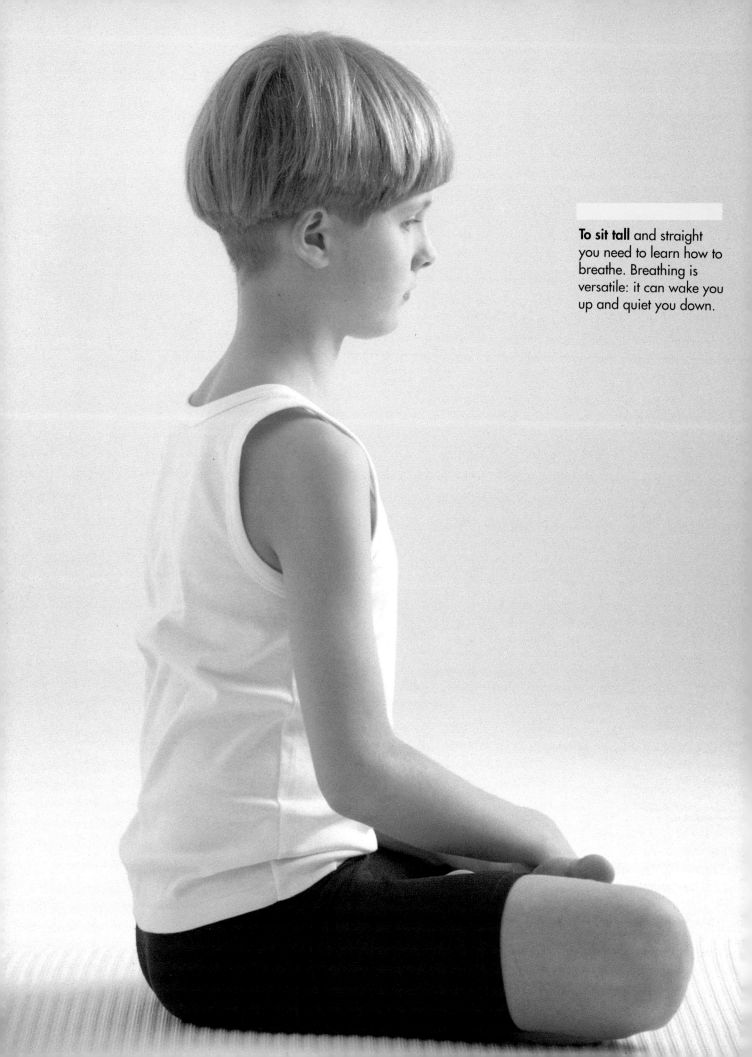

To sit tall and straight you need to learn how to breathe. Breathing is versatile: it can wake you up and quiet you down.

USING YOUR BREATH

Yawning, buzzing, blowing, hissing and Lion pose are enjoyable ways to help you learn how to breathe quietly and evenly. They all involve using your breath in different ways. Feel how they affect your shoulders, your hips and your stomach.

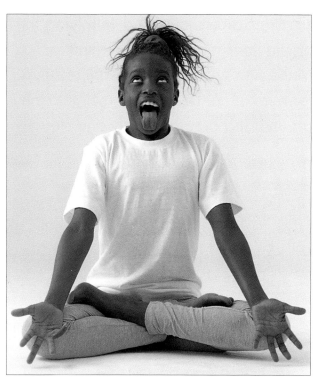

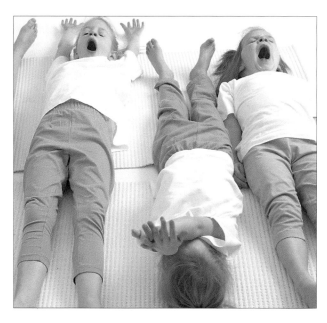

Yawning (*left*) means taking a big breath as you stretch. Blowing (*below*) shows how long you can breathe out. Go steadily so the blowing is as strong at the end as at the beginning. For Lion (*above*) sit tall and straight. Breathe out through your mouth, stretch out your tongue, and look upwards.

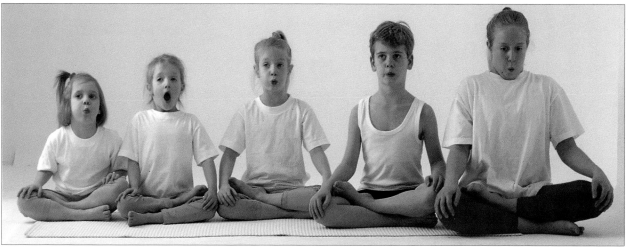

LYING FLAT

Savasana

Yoga practice should end with lying flat
on the floor for at least five minutes.
Make sure you are in the right position
for relaxation. Let yourself melt into the
ground and breathe slowly and steadily.

1 Lie flat on your back
with your knees bent
up. Cross your arms over
your chest so that your
back lies flat. Stay for a
minute. Your head, hips
and shoulders should be
in line. Hugging Teddy is
optional, but you should
really keep your head
centred.

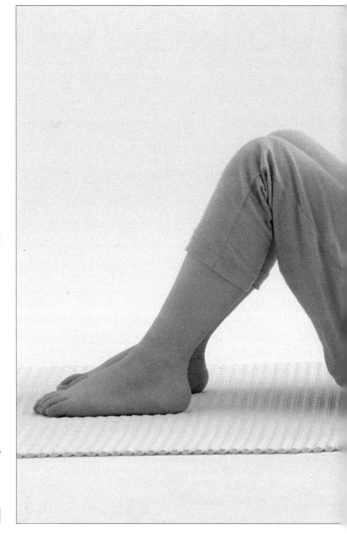

2 After lying with your
knees bent up,
breathe out and stretch
out your legs. Let your
arms flop to the floor
beside you, palms facing
up. Feel your body really
heavy on the ground and
sink down further every
time you breathe out. This
position is known as
Dead Man's pose.

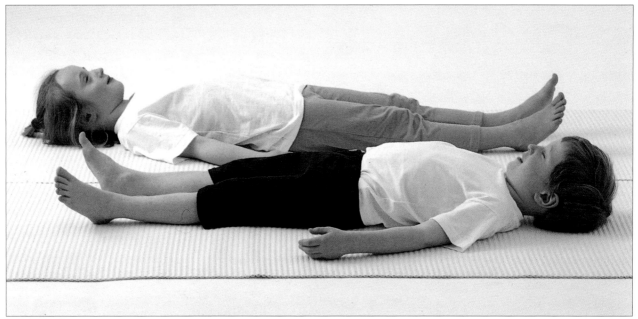

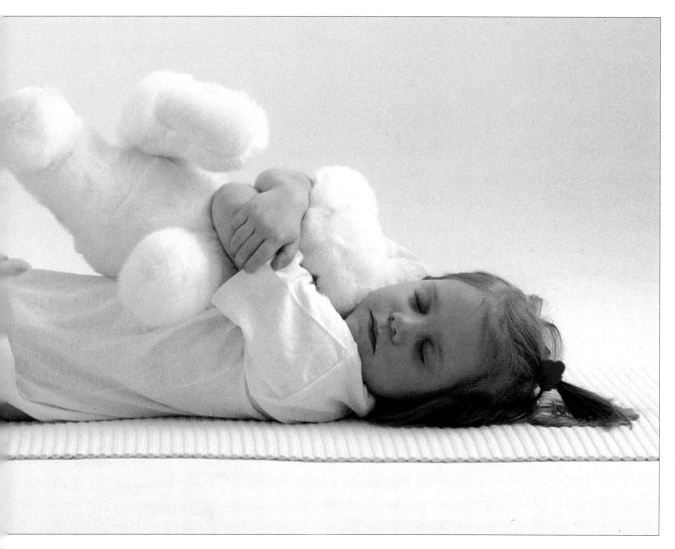

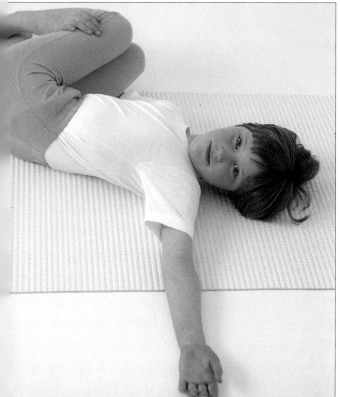

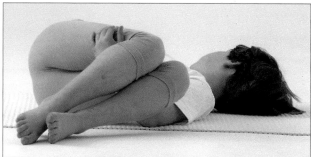

Lying Twist This simple stretch can be done before you relax or as a stretch at the end before you get up off the floor. Lie flat on your back with your knees bent up.

Breathe out and flop your knees and hips to one side and let your head roll over to the other. Come back to the center and do the same on the other side.

97

PLAY

Yoga should always be fun. Then the body will simply let go spontaneously. This is a magical ability natural to children and all too quickly lost as they get older.

When they have been exercising in a group, children will need a chance to let off steam as well as be quiet. But fun does not have to involve competition or showing off. The games on the following pages include the poses learned throughout the book. Parents can enjoy playing them with their children at home. And they provide a stimulating way to end a class before it is time to quiet down.

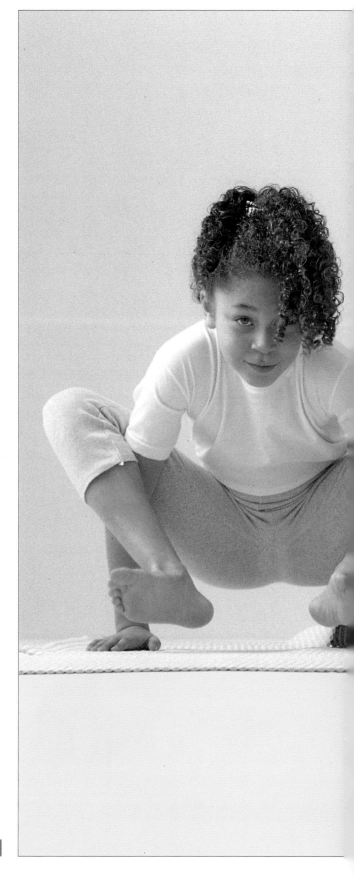

Sometimes it takes time to get the poses right. It can be fun trying to do them in a group even if, as here, there are more fallen birds than flying ones (page 38).

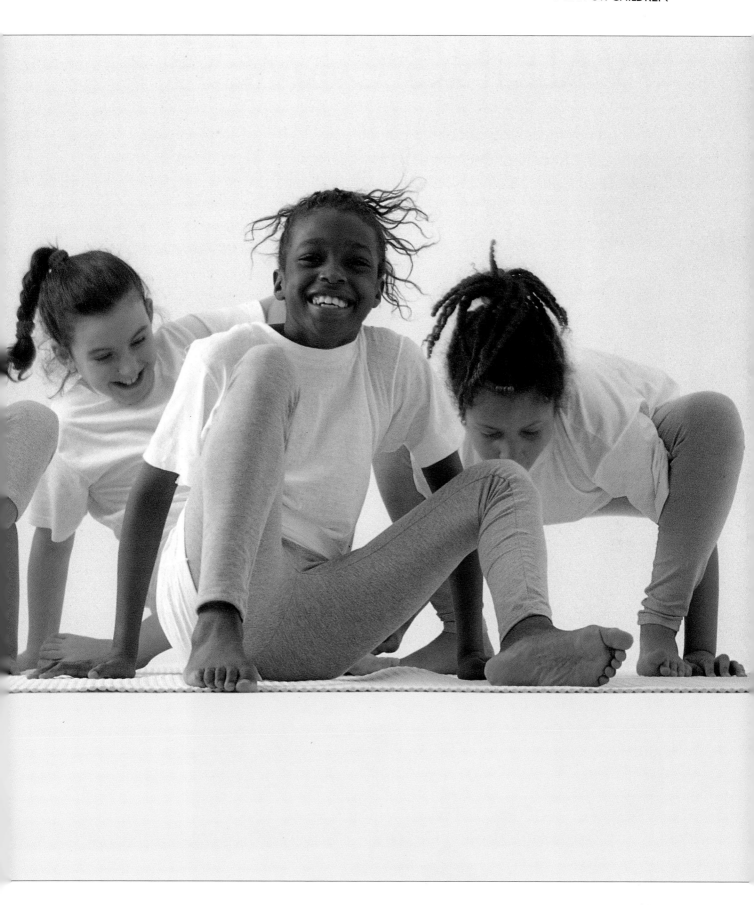

WALKING GAMES

These games teach you about the pull of gravity - the force that anchors us to the earth. They make you feel as if your feet are glued to the ground. This helps your spine stretch and grow tall.

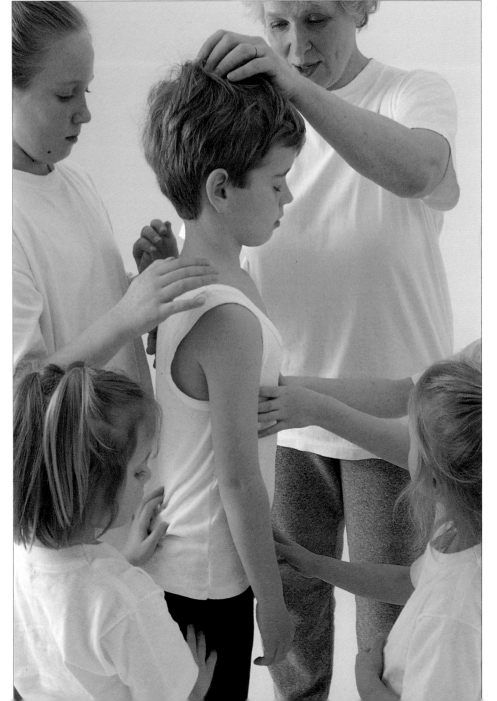

Gravity Game You stand in a small circle with one child in the center. You all then help the child in the middle. If you're the one in the center stand straight with feet immovable and let yourself fall forwards, sideways, or backwards as the other children, standing very close, catch you. Eventually you will find your straight, effortless, standing balance. Then it's someone else's turn.

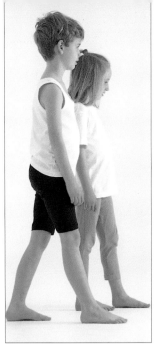

Giants Walking Stand as if you had huge heavy boots on (left). Walk slowly imagining that it is almost impossible to take your back foot off the floor because it is so heavy. Stretch tall as you walk. Still with the feet heavy, turn as you walk so that you stretch even further. When your back foot is really heavy you can go all the way into Triangle pose (page 24) and Standing Twist (page 26) as you walk. Perhaps this is how the original giants grew so tall. The heavier their feet, the more they stretched as they walked.

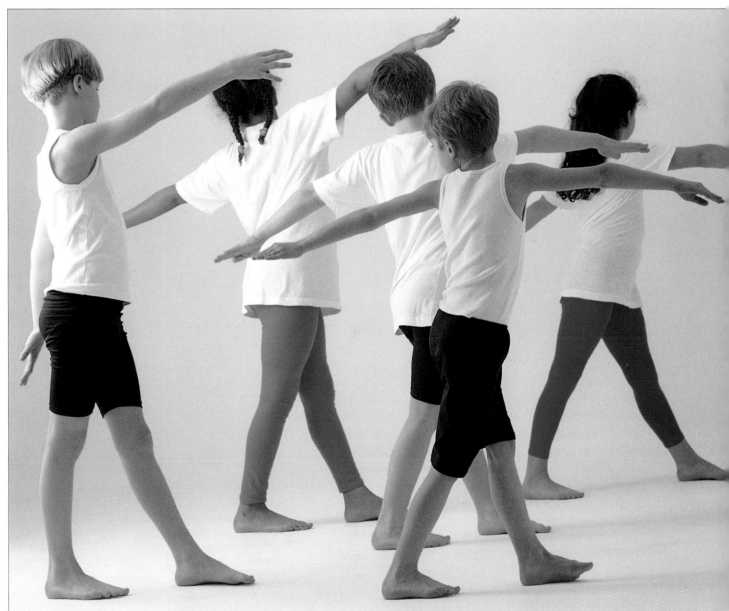

ANIMAL GAMES

Many yoga poses are named after animals. You can make up games using the characteristics of each animal.

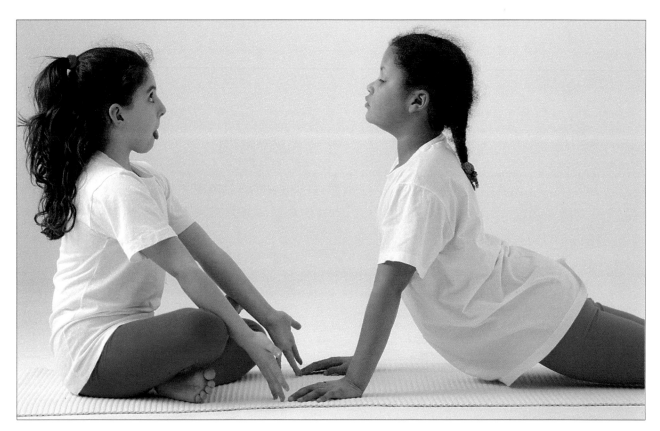

Lion, Mouse and Snake
Pairs of children close their eyes, then each child silently decides whether to be a Lion (page 95), Snake (page 66) or Mouse (page 82). They win or lose depending on what the other half of the pair chooses to be: the snake wins over the mouse because it can eat him, but loses against the lion which can crush him; the mouse can escape from the lion but loses to the snake; the lion loses against the mouse but wins over the snake. Once they are in the poses, someone gives the word and they open their eyes to see who's won. If they choose the same pose three times running, they both get a prize.

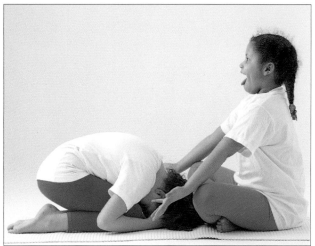

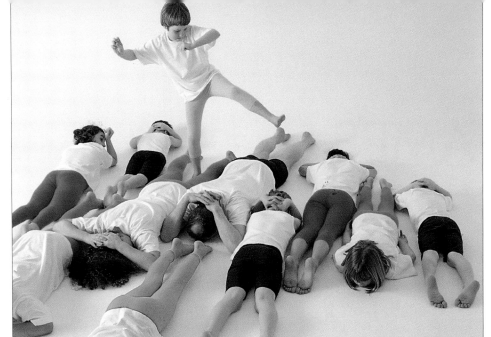

Crocodile Game All the children except one lie face down on the floor - they are logs floating down the river except that one is a crocodile in disguise. The child tries to cross the river safely. If the crocodile is touched it rears up in Crocodile pose ready to bite.

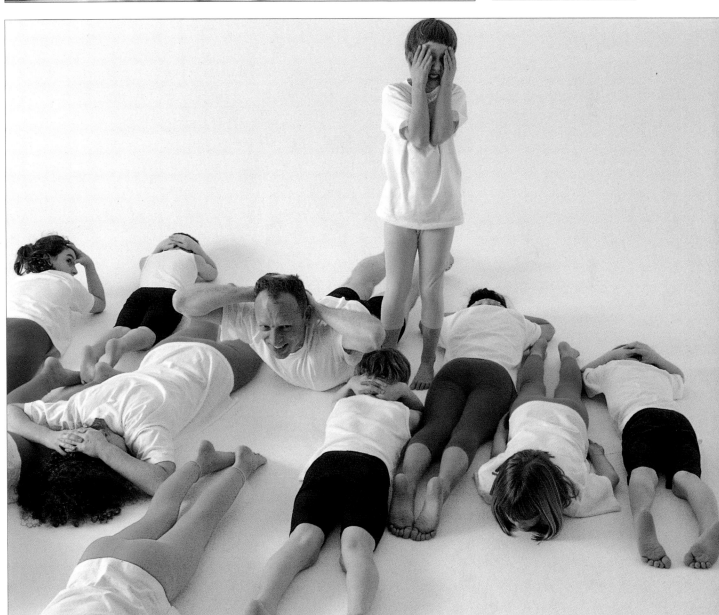

BALL GAMES

Yoga poses can be adapted to make simple ball games to be played either in a large group or with one or two children. Try throwing and catching in sitting or standing poses (*opposite*), or more elaborate games such as bowling.

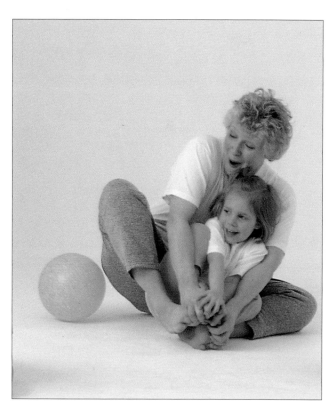

Bowling All the children except one sit in Butterfly pose (page 44) spaced out an arm's length away from each other - these are the bowling pins. The remaining child rolls a large ball towards the pins trying to knock them over. If you're hit or you come out of Butterfly, you're out of the game.

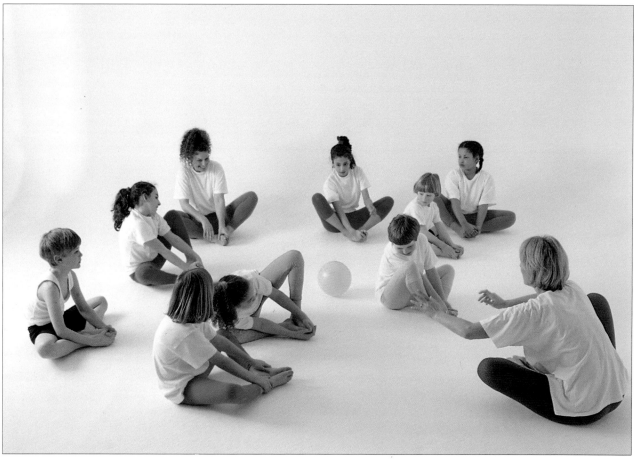

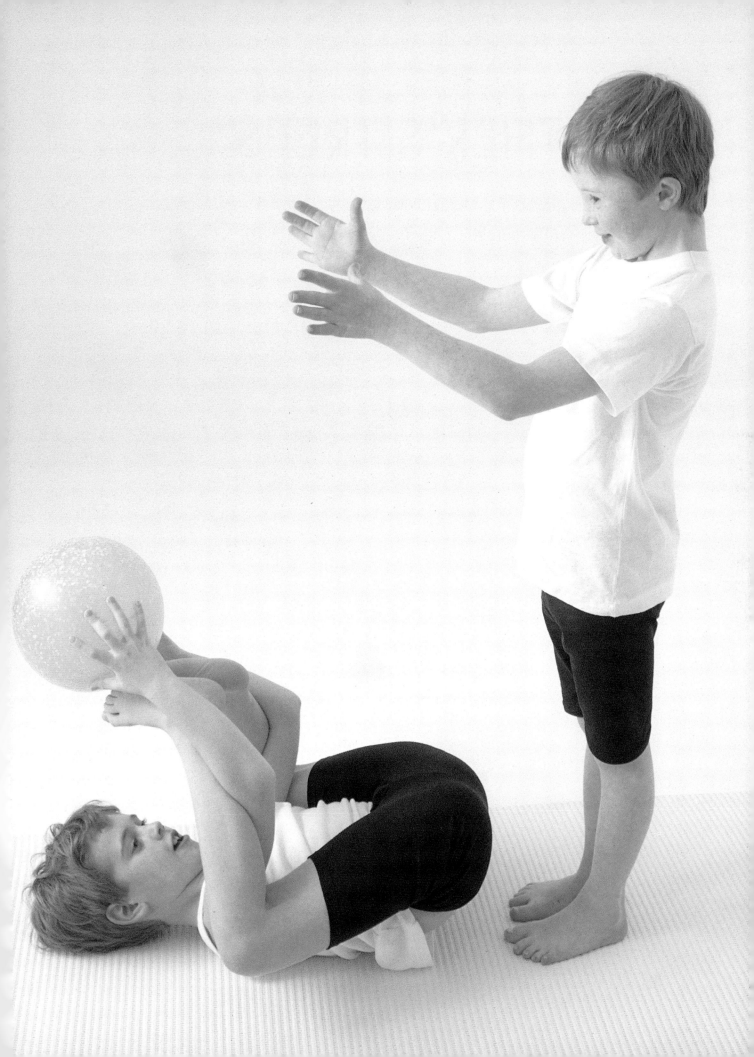

PLAY

MOTHER'S TREES

This game is played like Mother May I, but as well as creeping up on mother the players practice Tree pose.

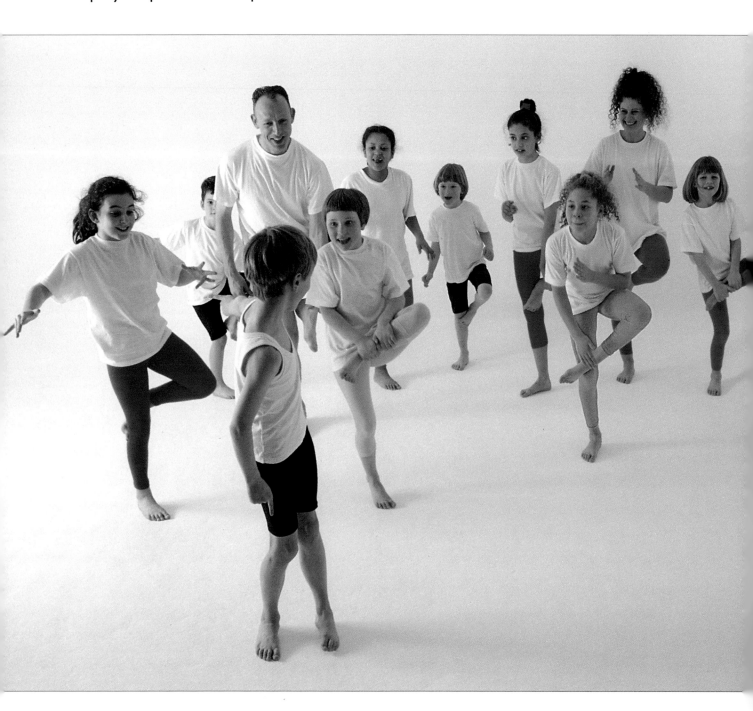

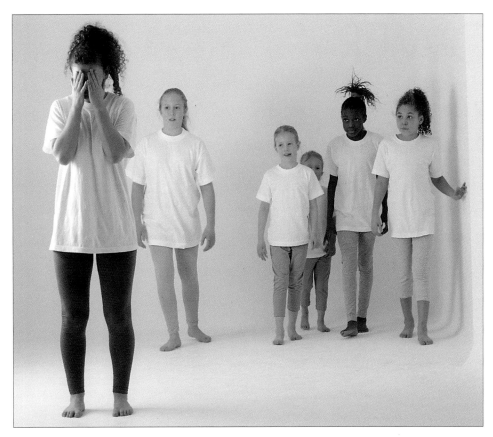

One child is elected to be 'mother'. The rest of the children all start at the back of the room and try to creep up on her. When mother turns around suddenly they all freeze in Tree pose (page 18). Swaying about is allowed but anyone caught with both feet on the floor has to go to the back and start again. The first to reach mother and touch her takes her place.

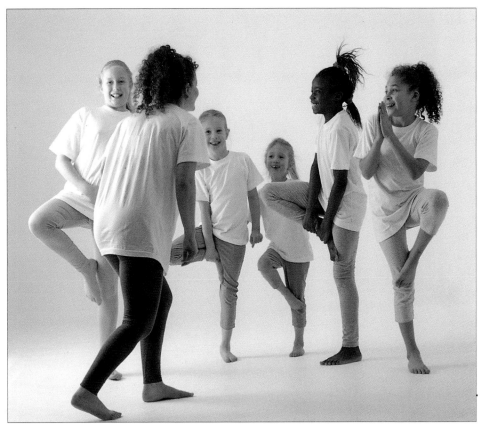

SUNFLOWER

The Sundance (page 72) done by a circle of children makes a sunflower. You need at least six children and, to make a proper flower with all the petals opening out at the same time, everyone has to stay together. Wait for each other. Don't race ahead.

Stand in a circle facing inwards with your palms together (as in step 1 of Sundance). Then continue in the sequence: breathe in and stretch up; breathe out and flop forward into Rag Doll; breathe in and take the left leg back; breathe out, take the other leg back and go into Dog pose; if you need to rest here, bend your knees and do Mouse (*below*) letting the flower fold its petals and go to sleep; then breathe in and out again and go down flat, breathe in and do Snake (*right*); finally, breathe out and go back into Dog. Now reverse the sequence right back to the beginning. Take it slowly and steadily throughout.

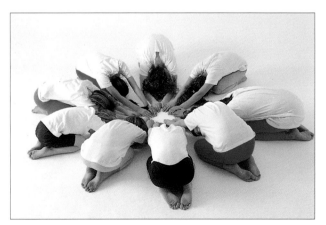

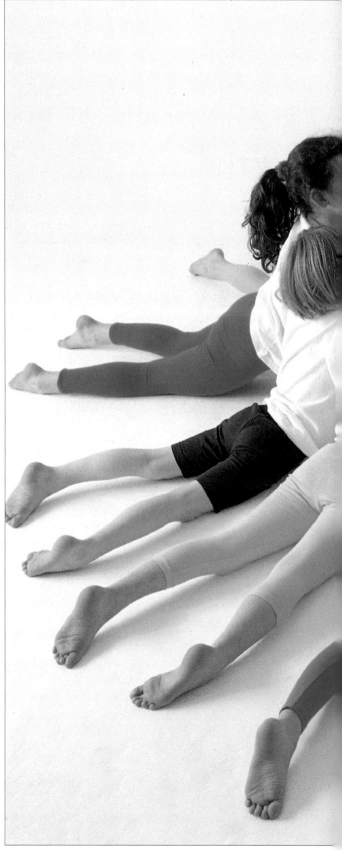

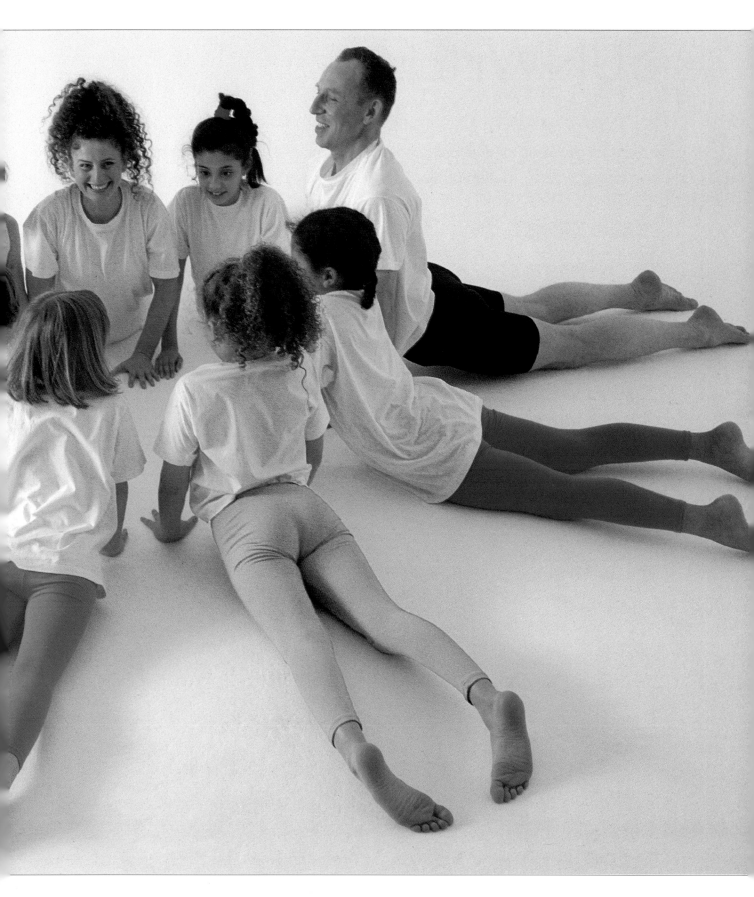

SUNWHEEL

This circle game can be played with a very large group of children with one large circle inside the other.

It can also be played with as few as four. Very small children particularly enjoy doing this with grown-ups.

1 Sit in a circle with your legs wide apart and your feet touching the person on each side of you so that the circle is closed. Place your hands on your legs. One person calls out 'left' or 'right' or 'center'.

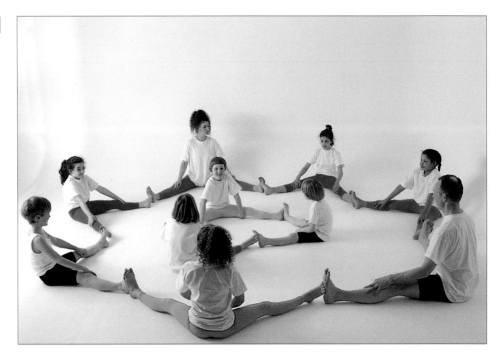

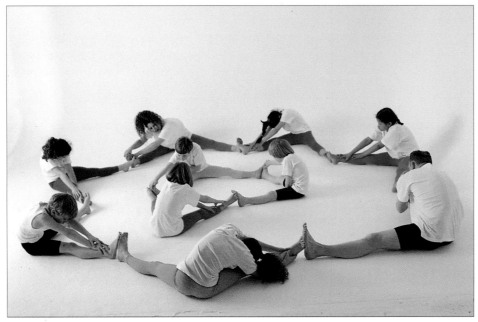

2 When you go to the right, stretch over to your right and try to catch your right foot.

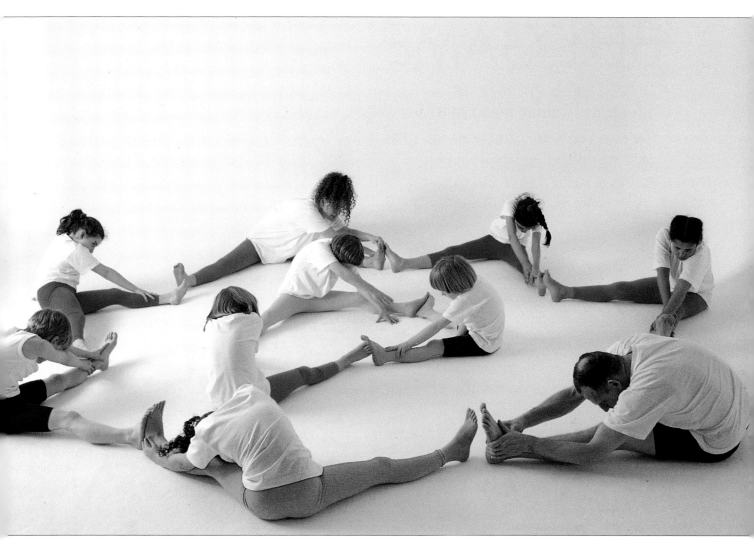

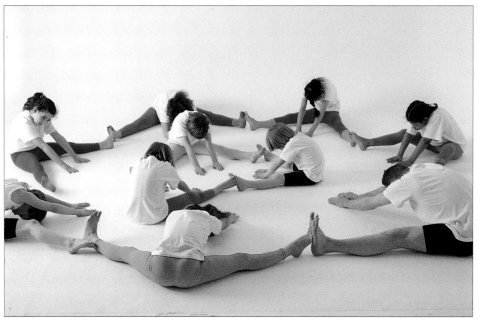

3 When you go to the left stretch over to your left and try to catch your left foot.

4 When you go to the center stretch forward from your hips and stretch your hands to the center.

BELL GAME

This game is about being quiet yet alert. You need at least six children to play it well. You also need a small bell.

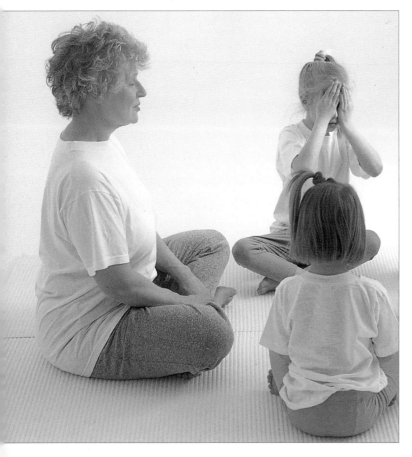

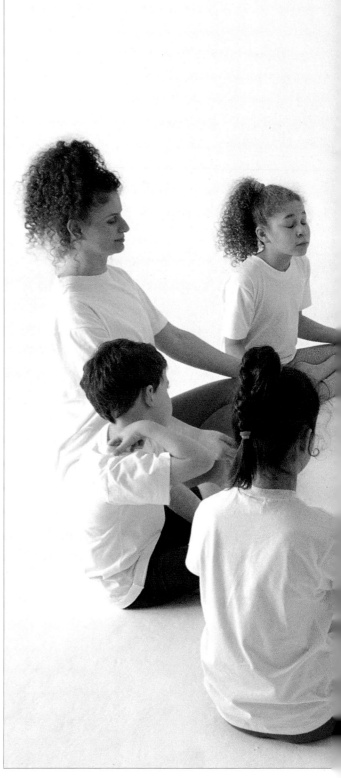

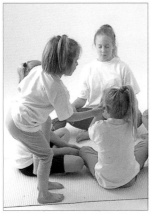

1 Sit everyone in a circle facing inwards with their eyes closed. Choose one person to start the game. He or she tiptoes very softly around the outside of the circle and rings a small bell very gently near the ear of the person of their choice.

2 The two change places. And so it goes on. At the end of the game when eyes are opened, the circle is still intact but everyone has changed places.

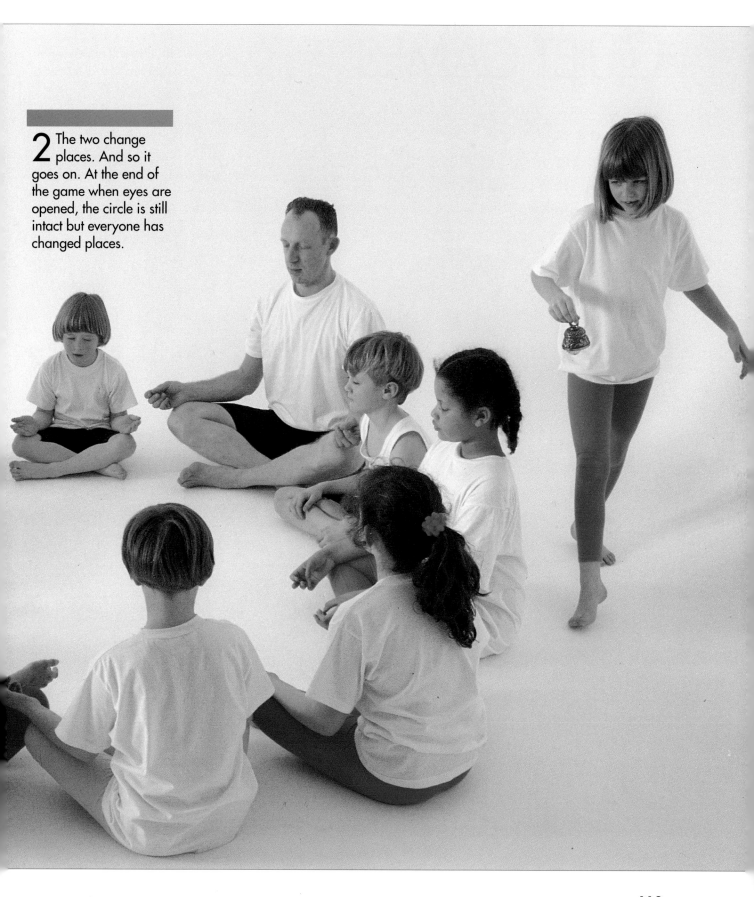

QUIET GAMES

It can be fun to sit quietly with friends in a yoga group. You will discover how to breathe evenly and calmly; and learn to become aware of one another's breathing.

Sit very tall and straight with your backs touching each other all the way up, the backs of your heads touching, too. Feel each other breathing through your backs. Breathe in and out slowly in time with each other. Sit as still as you can.

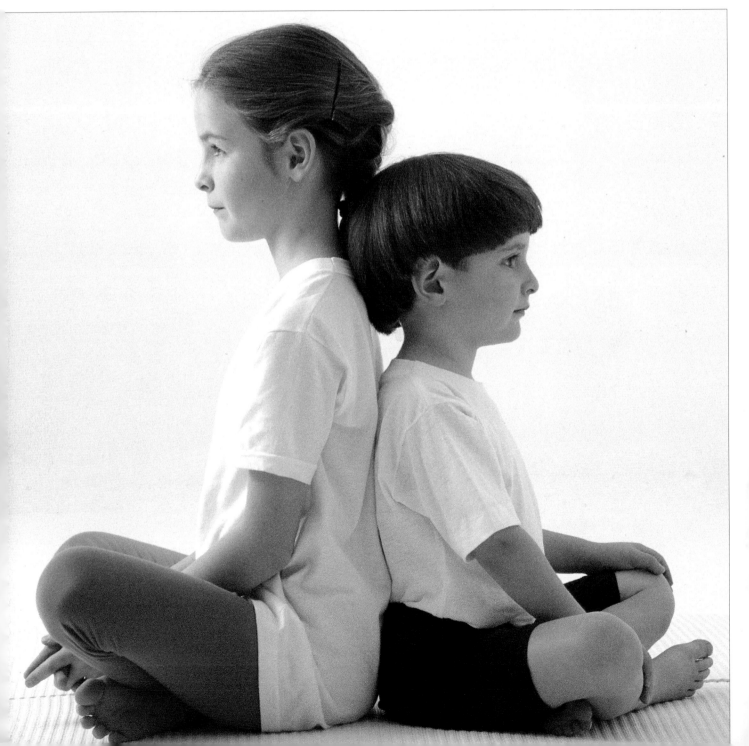

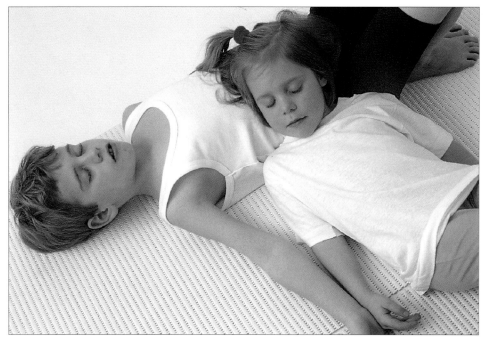

Breathing Snake This is something a whole group of children can do together. Everybody lies on the floor with knees bent up, each child's head on someone else's abdomen. You can feel the abdomen move up as the breath goes in and move down as the breath goes out.

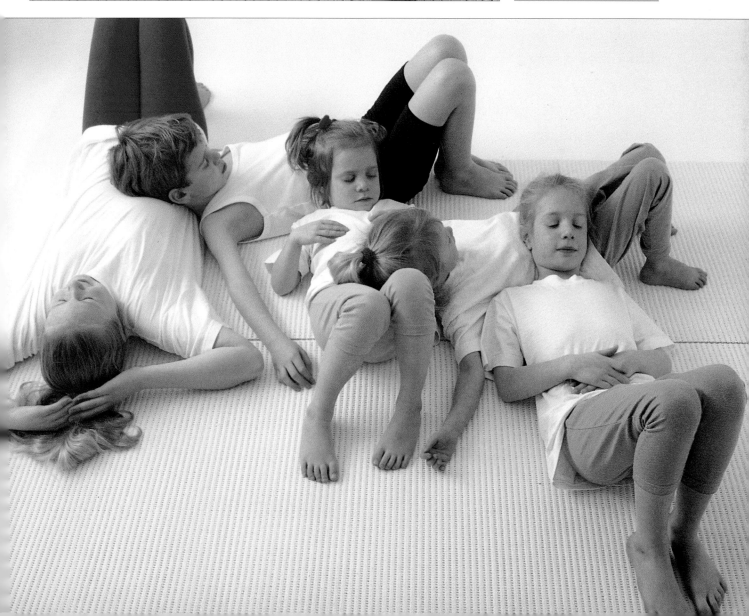

NEEDS

To a certain extent everyone has special needs. All children are individuals. Their bodies and minds are different. Their abilities, their strengths and weaknesses are different. Even otherwise healthy and active children can develop bad habits of sitting, standing and movement which will cause problems later on if uncorrected. Some sporting activities can develop imbalances of posture and coordination. For disabled children such difficulties are, of course, much more intense.

In this chapter familiar problem areas are highlighted - spine, shoulders, hips, feet - and simple ways to restore flexibility are suggested.

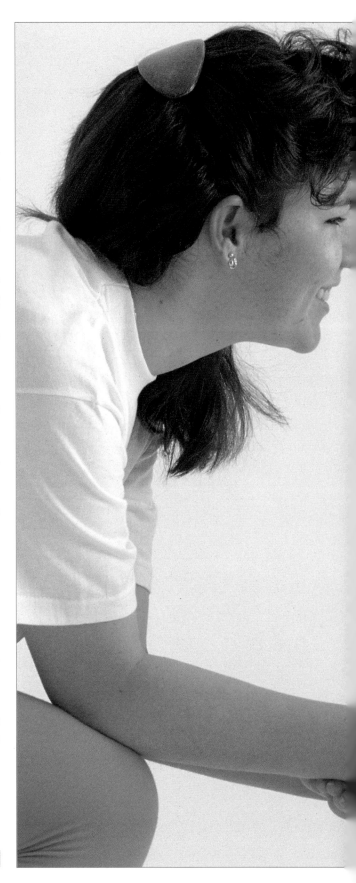

A child with no movement in her legs can be helped to flex her hips and stretch her lower back. In this version of Squat (page 30) she is using her hands to fold herself into the position.

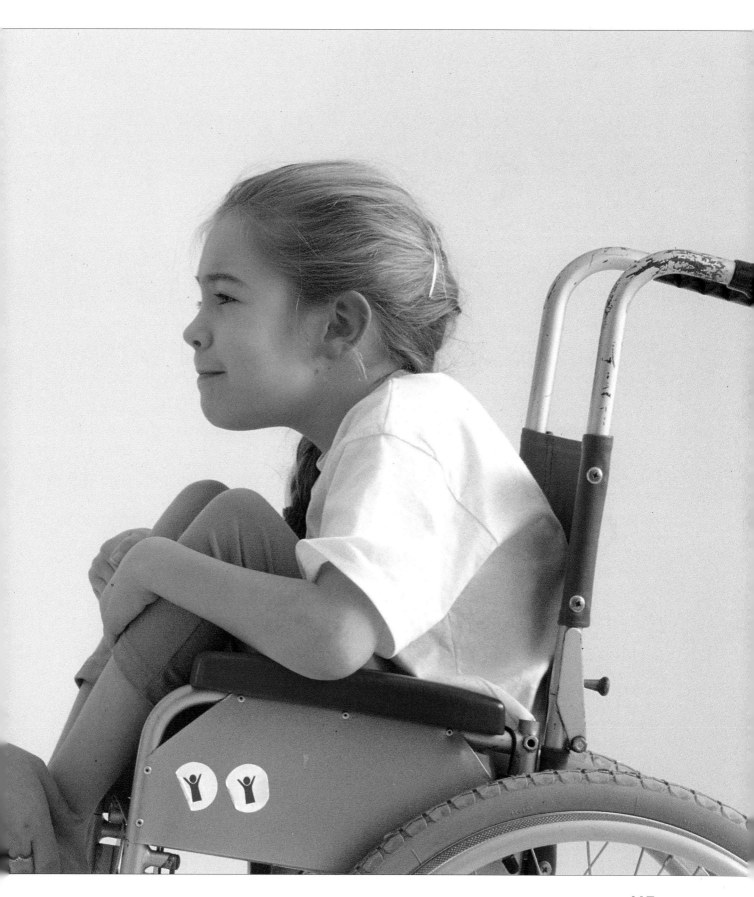

Yoga is essentially non-competitive. There is no physical peak or goal to be reached, so children of widely differing physical abilities can enjoy doing it together.

Those whose physical potential falls outside the range considered normal are often prescribed exercises in the form of physiotherapy. Such exercises can become an unwelcome chore and seem to set them apart from other children. But disabled children can have just as much fun and derive as much benefit as other children in a yoga group, and they will not feel isolated from their friends. In fact, it can be surprising how some disabled children (such as the Down's syndrome boy on page 119) can be more flexible than their more able companions.

Imbalances of posture and coordination, stiffness and tension in back and joints can affect children as young as six years old, and they may well need to do exercises to correct these problems. Others may need to redress the effects of overextending themselves in sporting activities.

PROBLEM AREAS

Back Parents of young babies watch them constantly as they learn to walk, hovering anxiously and noticing every detail. Once a toddler is independently on the move, naturally, the careful supervision lessens, and bad habits begin to develop unnoticed.

Uneven sitting and lopsided games seem harmless at this stage but can gradually lead to back problems later. Even how you carry your baby and how it sits in its stroller are important. Doctors in the West are already questioning

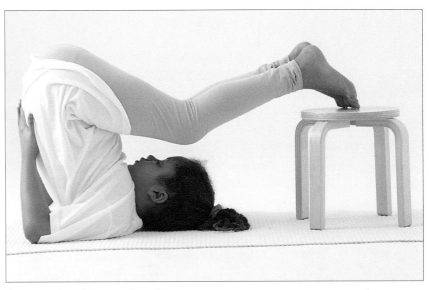

If you are stiff in Plow Pose , don't push yourself too far. Drop your legs over on to a stool.

the use of walkers and early rocking chairs for the same reasons.

Poses which specifically benefit the spine include all the standing poses (pages 16-31), Dog (page 32), Cat (page 34), Turtle (page 56), Plow (page 62), Locust (page 64), Snake (page 66), Bridge (page 68), Sundance (page 72) and Lying Twist (page 97).
Hips Children in Africa and Asia are often carried, with their legs apart, on their mothers' backs. They squat and sit cross-legged on the floor instead of on comfortable chairs and sofas. Such children maintain the full range of flexibility in their hip joints all their lives.

Lack of mobility in these areas can be restored by exercises such as Butterfly (page 44) and Hero (page 40) which work the hips in opposite directions. Also try Wigwam (page 28), Fan (page 50), Squat (page 30), Bird (page 36) and Cow (page 54).
Shoulders Round shoulders, stiff shoulders, right- and left-handedness, all affect the entire structure of the body and contribute towards it developing unevenly. In extreme cases tension

in the upper body can affect the way you breathe. Stiffness in the shoulders can pull your head out of line and contribute to headaches. Crouching over school desks and computers for lengths of time all add up to later discomfort. Poses which will help restore mobility in shoulders include Cow (page 54), Dog (page 32) and Sundance (page 72). See also page 120.
Feet Because feet are composed of many small bones, it's easy for the arches to drop and become distorted. This is one of the main reasons why shoes - if they must be worn at all at an early age - need to be carefully chosen for width and support. For flexible feet sit on your heels with your toes tucked under (page 86, step 4) - it's much more difficult than you might think. Also practice pointing and lifting each toe individually (see also page 121).
Knees Stiffness in the knee joints can be eased by practicing the upside down poses such as Candle and Scissors (pages 60-62). In

these poses the knees are stretched straight but there is no weight on them. Sitting in Fan (page 50) is also helpful.

SPORTING PROBLEMS

Sports and games are fine as long as care is taken to counteract the effects of one-sided or repetitive movements. Few sports or exercise programs are concerned to work each joint and muscle of the body evenly. Many encourage one-sided development in order to reach a standard of excellence in one particular area. Yoga can help counteract such extremes.

The tennis player, for example, needs to work the opposite side of the body to the stroke arm in poses like Cow (page 54), Triangle (page 24) and Bow and Arrow (page 52). The breaststroke swimmer would benefit from Dog (page 32), Back-bends such as Wheel (page 70), and Candle poses (page 60) to redress the balance.

The skier needs Fan (page 50), Wigwam (page 28) and Locust (page 64) or Snake (page 66) to stretch out straight after a long run.

For taking part in one-sided

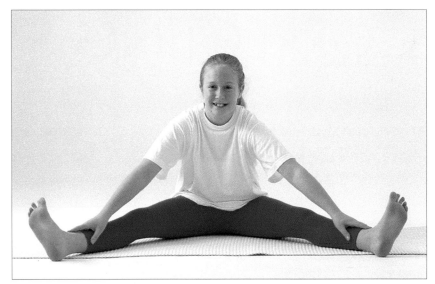

sports such as golf, fencing, hockey, baseball and all the racquet games, Cow (page 54) and Sundance (page 72) are helpful. Practice the pose twice on the underused arm side.

Runners and footballers need to stretch out their hamstrings. Rag Doll (page 22), Plow with a stool (page 63), and Dog (page 32) are good for this.

DISABILITIES

Some children's problems start earlier in life, from conception or at birth, or have arisen through

Sitting up straight in Fan pose stretches the hamstrings and knees.

accident or illness. These children fall outside the range of what is usually considered to be normal and their needs are more extreme than the average child. For this book, two children, one who has cerebral palsy and one Down's syndrome were able to enjoy working in a yoga group. Obviously, such children need extra attention during group practice and the teacher should always check with their doctor beforehand. Yoga poses can usually be practiced alongside other therapeutic regimes.

In the following pages are poses which are specifically suitable for wheelchairbound children.

Some children - such as some of those with Down's syndrome - suffer from hypermobility. Yoga is ideal for such children as it encourages coordination and stability as well as allowing them to enjoy and be admired for their flexibility without overextending.

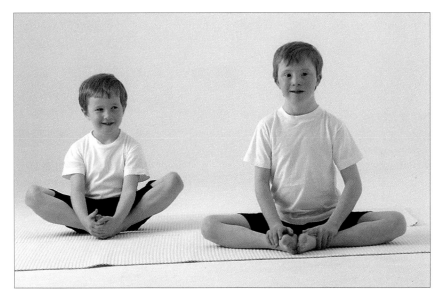

A boy with Down's syndrome is more flexible than his little brother.

CORRECTING STIFFNESS

Some children are much stiffer than others and, for them, small precise movements are helpful. On these pages common problem areas are tackled and some simple ways to correct them are suggested.

Prayer pose is very helpful for stiff shoulders. Place your palms together, fingers pointing down. Breathe out and turn your hands so that they are pointing upward. Try to get your hands as far up your back as possible while keeping all the fingers touching each other.

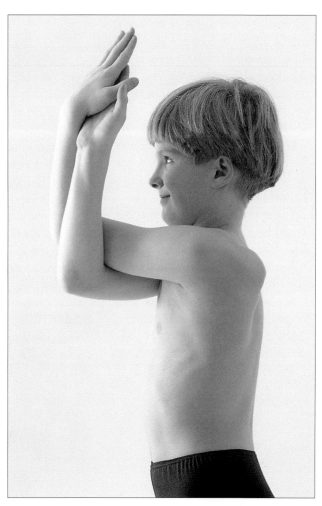

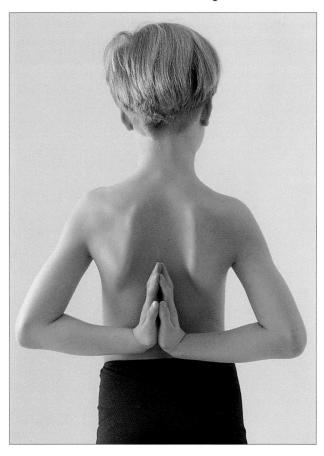

Half Eagle This is also good for shoulders. Cross your left elbow over your right one, then wrap your lower arms around each other so that the palms are facing.

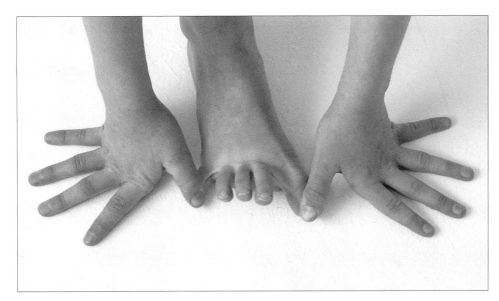

Feet Make sure that all your toes can spread out and that the arches of your feet are strong. Practice lifting up your middle three toes while your big and little toes stay on the floor. If this is impossible for you, hold your outer toes down to begin with.

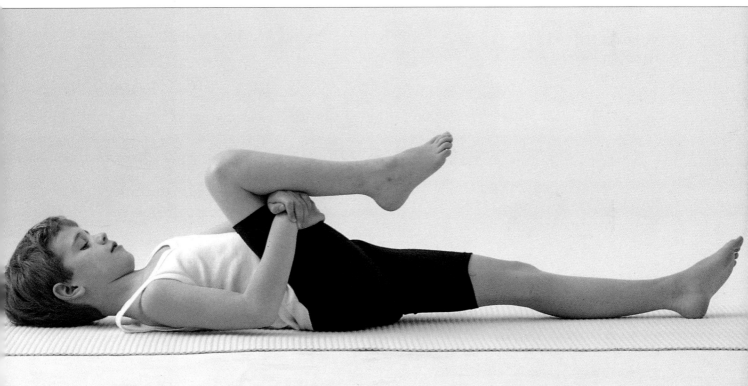

Hips and Lower Back
This knee to chest pose helps to increase flexibility in the hips and lower back. Lie on your back and hug one knee towards you as you breathe out. The other leg stretches away from you along the floor. Repeat with the other leg.

121

CHAIR POSES

Many yoga poses can be adapted for chairbound children. Of course, what they can do will depend on the nature of their disability. A child in a wheelchair may need help in any of these positions.

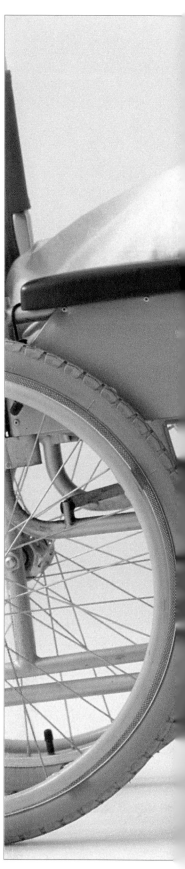

Legs Up Sit tall and then, as you breathe out, hug one knee close to your chest. Stay for a couple of breaths and then repeat on the other side. Then try both legs.

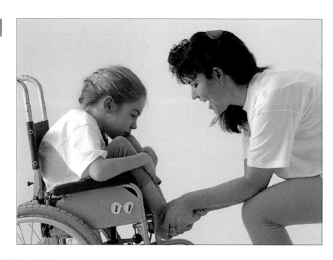

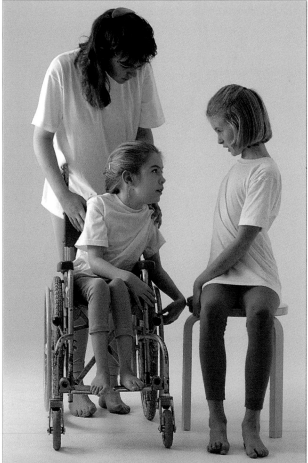

Sitting Twist Sit up as tall as you can (*left*), turn. Keep hips down and knees facing forwards, and turn your shoulders as far around to one side as possible. Repeat on the other side.

Rag Doll Sit as straight as you can. Breathe out, flop forward and touch your feet (*right*). For a child in a wheelchair making an effort to keep their head and shoulders up, this pose is a welcome antidote to tension.

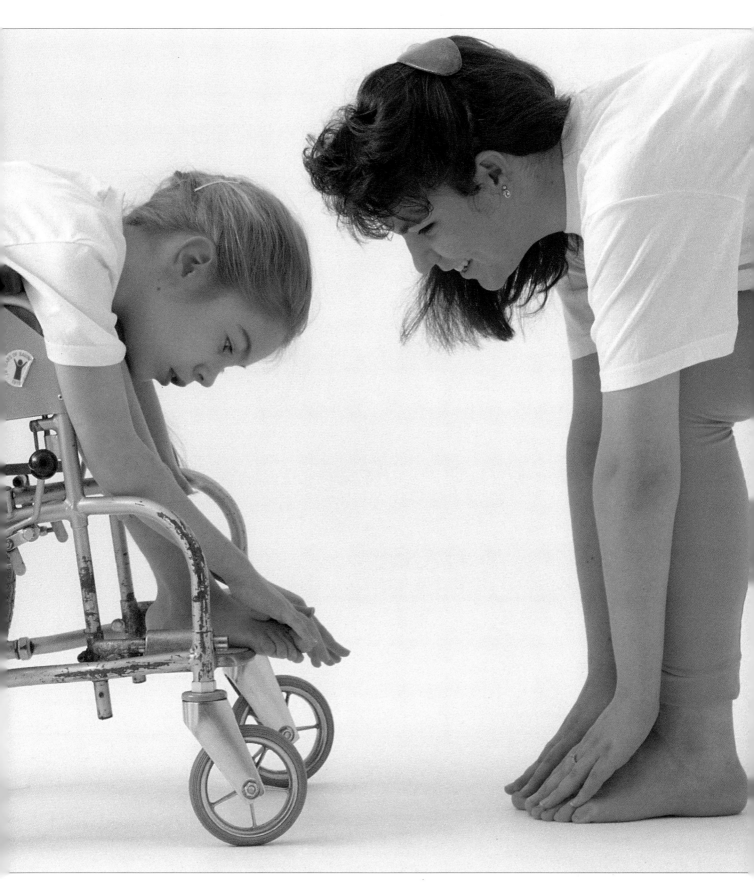

FLOOR POSES

Disabled children enjoy exercizing on the floor with others. Every child's abilities vary so it's important to find out what the disabled child can and can't do. One of the girls in the pictures has cerebral palsy and cannot use her legs. These floor exercises are gentle and beneficial. Sitting games such as Bowling and Sunwheel (pages 104 and 110) could also be suitable.

Lying twist Lie on your back with knees bent up and arms out. Children who spend much of their time in a wheelchair will need help initially to lie straight. Breathe out and let the knees and hips flop over to one side. Turn your head in the opposite direction. Stay like this for a minute or two breathing deeply and letting your back lengthen. Come back to the middle and do the same pose on your other side.

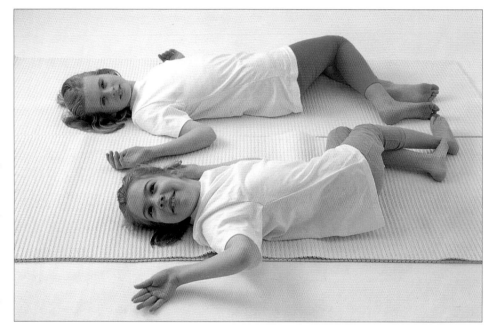

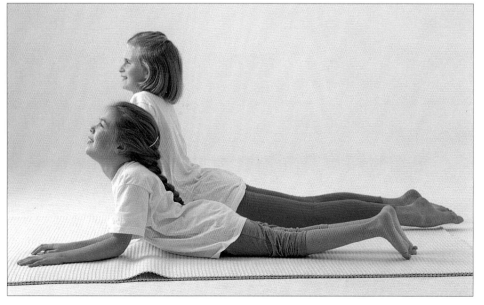

Modified snake Lie on your front with your arms bent beside you with the elbows and palms down. Let your elbows drop down heavily on to the floor. Breathe out and lift first your head and then as much of your chest as you can. Disabled children can do this on their own if helped to lie on the floor. The child here can curve up quite a long way.

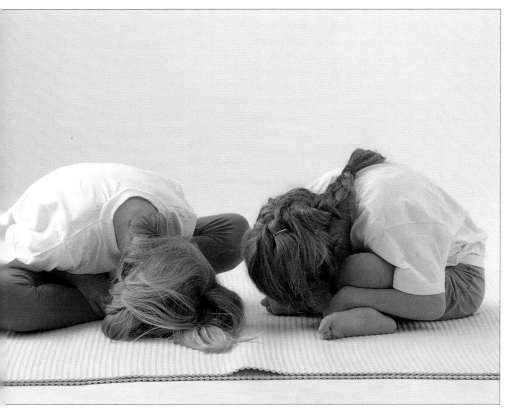

Forward bend Sit on the floor with your legs crossed. Let somebody help with this first stage. Your hips must stay firmly down on the floor. Then bend forwards as you breathe out. Breathe in and feel your back getting wider and then let it grow longer as you breathe out. Come up as you breathe out.

Rolling Just rolling between poses can provide exercise and fun.

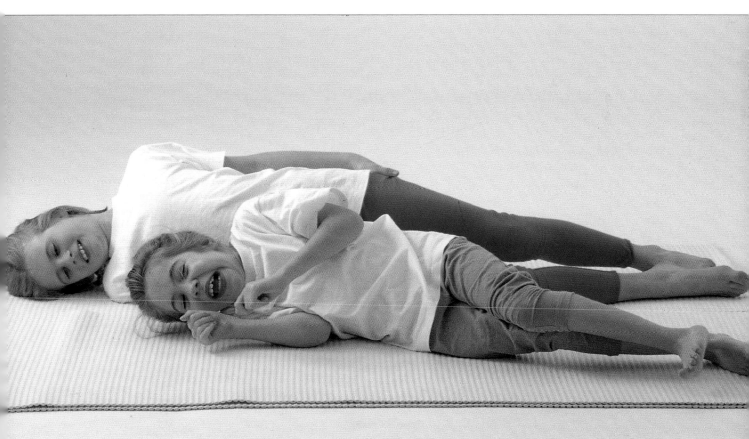

INDEX

ACKNOWLEDGEMENTS

The authors and publishers would like to thank all those who helped in the preparation of this book, in particular, the adults and children who took part in the photography sessions. The adults were Joy Anderson, Chloe Blegvad, John Glyn, Natasha McDougall and Lucy Su. The children were Elodene Baker, Louis Barron, Natasha Bernes, Beatrice and Olivia Boyle, Tiffany Ann Brew, Robin Bridge, Becky Butler, Kaye and Vigo Blegvad, Henrietta and Michael Dale, Louise Daley, Naomi Edmonds, Mia Gibson, Natasha Griffin, Caspar, Celia and Matthew Le Fanu, Stephanie and Pierre Moorsom, Oscar Pye-Jeary, Nico Shattock, Kate and Lucy Solomons, Hamish and Anna Stewart, Lucy and David Walsh, and Thea, Amelia and Vita Wrightson.

They would also like to thank Wendy Grace for her tireless help in transporting the children to and fro; Maeve Larkin for her friendly advice; Aram Associates for lending the Aalto stools used in some of the photographs; and, finally, Anthony Pye-Jeary for his endless patience and his cooking.

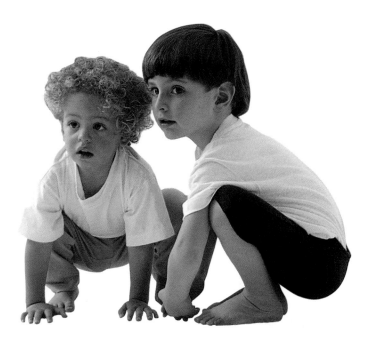

THE AUTHORS

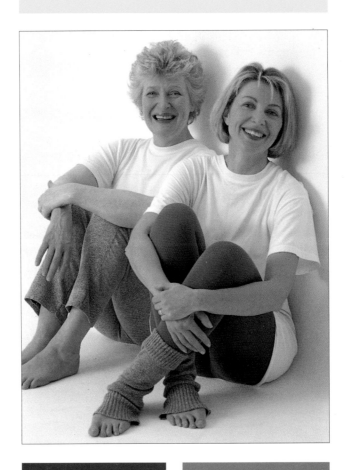

Mary Stewart has been teaching yoga for more than 20 years to private clients, classes and teachers of yoga all over the world. She has developed her own methods based on breathing, and believes that children, in particular, require a special approach. This is her fourth book.

Kathy Phillips is a journalist specializing in fashion and design. She contributes to British magazines and newspapers such as *Tatler, Mirabella*, the *Daily Mail, Daily Telegraph, Sunday Telegraph, Mail on Sunday* and *YOU Magazine*. She has been practicing yoga for more than 15 years.